Peter Mansfield practised for many years as a music teacher, before training to teach the Alexander Technique and the Bates Method of Vision Education. His book on the Bates Method has been widely acclaimed as a clear and authoritative guide to this often misunderstood subject. He has over fifteen years' experience of using Flower Remedies, both for personal benefit, and in conjunction with his Bates Method practice where clearing emotional issues is often an important part of the process of clearing vision.

Peter lives in Sussex where he divides his time between teaching, writing and dinghy sailing.

Also by Peter Mansfield:

THE BATES METHOD

ALTERNATIVE HEALTH

FLOWER REMEDIES

PETER MANSFIELD

Illustrated by Shaun Williams

OPTIMA

An OPTIMA Book

First published in Great Britain
by Optima in 1995

Copyright © Peter Mansfield 1995

The right of the author has been asserted.

ISBN 0–356–21050–2

Typeset by Solidus (Bristol) Limited
Printed and bound in Great Britain by
Clays Ltd, St. Ives PLC

Optima
A Division of
Little, Brown and Company (UK)
Brettenham House
Lancaster Place
London WC2E 7EN

Contents

Introduction

The main reason for writing this book was to find out things I wanted to know. The idea which eventually led to the commission to write it came originally from a conversation with Jayne Booth, my then editor, while we were preparing my first book *The Bates Method*. I was sharing with Jayne the importance that I attached to the use of the Bach remedies and some of the remarkable results I had had with them, and also the interest I felt in the developing 'new' remedies. Although she was generally well versed in natural healing methods, it was clear that a lot of this was new information as far as Jayne was concerned and I suggested that someone ought to write a book giving some sort of overview of the situation. She responded that I seemed to know more about it than anyone she had spoken to, and why didn't I take it on? So I started to make some enquiries and this book, rather later on, is the result.

Over the last 20 or so years a great revival of interest in flower essence therapy has led to the discovery or rediscovery and documentation of very large numbers of remedies by various people working in different locations and in different ways. Various schools of thought on the subject have ranged from those who regard all the 'new' remedies as bogus to the 'anything goes' approach of those who would prefer not to use anything developed longer ago than the last two weeks. In between are a lot of puzzled people who have perhaps heard vague rumours and contradictory opinions about one or more groups of essences but find it hard to locate information, or to fit it, when found, into any coherent scheme.

This was the position in which I found myself a few years ago. I had used the Bach Remedies® for many years with great success and was well aware not only of their power, but of the elegant subtlety and versatility of Dr Bach's system. When I began to hear of large numbers of new remedies emanating from, among other places, the west coast of the USA, my initial reaction was just a touch cynical, and that cynicism grew as the reports of ever more new families of remedies increased. At the same time, friends and colleagues – people whose judgement I respected – kept enthusing about the marvellous results they had achieved with these wonders – and so I began to explore.

The first part of the book is based on the Bach remedies, which for most people are still the best-known and most accessible form of flower therapy. The remainder sets out the results of my explorations, attempting to systematise the information available in a way which will help the assimilation of new information as it comes along. It can hardly pretend to be a definitive guide to the subject, since many of the known remedies are not documented anywhere, and more will, no doubt, remain to be discovered. But it will, I hope, point out some interesting directions: more of a 'backpacker's guide' than Baedecker's.

I have made full use of all the sources mentioned and have made the information section as comprehensive and accurate as possible so I hope that after reading this book, if you have not used flower remedies before you will know where to start, and if you are familiar with the 'old' remedies but have not known where to begin with the new, you will have an idea where to look for what you need to know.

PM

1

Principles of flower therapy

Before we can talk about healing, by whatever means, we need to have some idea of what we mean by sickness and health, and this, in turn, means that we need some definite idea about what we understand by 'life'. Modern physical medicine is very clever at manipulating the behaviour of the body in various ways, but it is less good at expressing what it finally expects to achieve.

We are beings of energy. Biology and the other 'life sciences' have concentrated almost exclusively on the study of chemical processes in living organisms, but these chemical processes are themselves only the grosser manifestations of energetic processes. Ancient philosophies have always described life in terms of pure energy and with each passing year, the discoveries of physicists make it clearer that this was no fanciful speculation but simple, sober truth, however hard it may be to see with the usual tools at our disposal. The matter of the body, like all matter, is

1

actually composed of patterns of energy, and all the processes of the body, in health as well as in sickness, are ultimately directed by the subtle movements and changes in those patterns.

PHYSICAL MEDICINE AND ENERGY MEDICINE

Physical medicine works directly on the body, aiming to alter the *results* of those movements and changes, but there are also various forms of *energy medicine* which aim to transform the patterns directly – homoeopathy, acupuncture, kinesiology, healing and meditation all work on this level, using different techniques to stimulate the body in the direction of greater balance and the removal of *dis-ease*.

All forms of energy medicine presuppose the existence of a *life energy* or *vital force* which sustains and organises the life of the physical body. Practitioners of physical medicine and physical scientists have disputed the existence of such a force, because they are unable to measure it. In fact, its existence is proven by the very existence of life. The laws of thermodynamics state that energy will always diffuse towards a state of equilibrium (heat will always pass from a hotter body to one which is cooler and cannot pass in the opposite direction) – the principle of *entropy*. A living body, however, defies entropy by concentrating energy in itself, drawing it in from the surroundings, and although various parts of the process can be described in terms of chemical reactions and so forth, no one has really answered in 'scientific' terms the question: what is it that holds living organisms together? Life energy or vital force is simply a label we can apply to the *something* that occupies that place. We do not know what it is or how it works, we can only know that if it did not exist, neither would we.

Most esoteric systems of healing describe an energy body

which forms a cocoon around the physical shape, controlling its development and growth. The physical body is seen as a secondary manifestation of this primary energy body, in the same way that the light which comes from a light bulb is a secondary manifestation of the (invisible) current flowing through the wires.

It is well known that the drugs and treatments of conventional allopathic medicine can do as much harm as good, which is why their dispensing is put into the hands of highly trained and regulated specialists. It is often asked whether this is not also true of so-called 'natural' medicines or, if not, how these remedies can possibly have the power to do any good?

Although understandable, this question is entirely wrong headed, because it fails to understand that the energy remedies are working in a completely different way. Allopathic medicine can be justified on one of two basic assumptions. The traditional idea, which has considerable merit, is that the body is naturally healthy and that sickness is caused by invasion by germs or other agencies. Ideally, the body defends itself against these invasions, indeed the only true cure is for the body to heal itself. The curative process can be helped by rest and suitable nursing care, providing the body with favourable conditions. If the invasion is too strong, overwhelming the defences and threatening death, medicines are used to hold the fort, while the body gathers its strength. The only problem is to find medicines and calculate doses which do more damage to the 'enemy' than to the body itself. Since both are living organisms this is tricky, to say the least, but doctors and patients both assume that it can and must be done.

This model still survives to inform a great deal of good conventional practice, but in other areas another more radical assumption seems to have taken hold, although it is

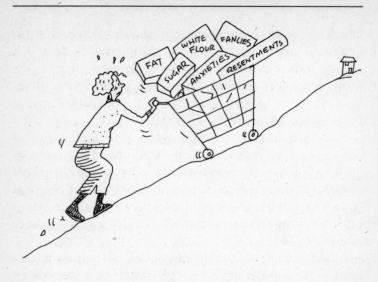

IT'S KEEPING THE BODY UNHEALTHY THAT
REQUIRES A GREAT DEAL OF FORCE
AND EFFORT...

never described explicitly. This is that the nature of the
body is to be unhealthy, or at least its tendency to health is
so unreliable that health and life can only be maintained by
more or less constant medical attention. (One symptom of
this way of thinking is that in official statistics, the 'health'
of a society is quantified in terms of the value of drugs
consumed and the expenditure on medical services.) In
other words, our bodies are subject to the laws of entropy,
constantly wanting to fall apart and only science and drugs
can push them back together. The action of allopathic
drugs applies a great deal of force to the body, with the
intention of making it better of course, but it is clear that
if sufficient force is applied a body can be made to do
anything at all, for good or ill, which is one reason why the

allopathic drugs can cause sickness as well as 'cure' it.

This second assumption is clearly wrong: in fact, the natural tendency of the body must be towards life and health, otherwise we would all die out in no time at all, to say nothing of the various millions of other life forms which have evolved and survived for millions of years without the benefit of scientific medicine. It is keeping the body *unhealthy* that requires a great deal of force and effort. Allowing the body to return to health obviously requires that this force is withdrawn: if this is done then change can be brought about by a very small stimulus, but only in the natural direction, just as a stone which can only be pushed uphill by brute force can be dislodged by a very small movement and will then roll downhill under its own energy.

VIBRATIONAL MEDICINE

The term *vibrational medicine* has been coined to describe work which aims to give such a stimulus, using the different energy patterns present in nature to modify the vibrations within living bodies, leading indirectly to changes on the physical plane. This encompasses on the one hand, methods which use the vibrations directly – light, sound, magnetism, etc. – and on the other, methods which involve the preparation of *essences* from the source of the vibration, which can then be absorbed into the body.

The most important and numerous of these are the flower and plant essences which are the main concern of this book, but the same principle can be applied to other sources of natural energy and we can also look at the essences prepared from those.

Why essences?

Liquids are generally the most sensitive carriers of vibrations. Sound travels further under water than through air and dropping a stone in a pond has a greater effect than dropping it on the ground. The flower preserved in a dry form would lose most of the vibrational quality which is preserved in the liquid essence. The human body is, we are told, composed largely of water, and it follows that for anything to be absorbed into the body, it needs to be in liquid form. The digestive tract exists largely to liquefy any food taken in so that its nutritional essence can be extracted and it is well understood that foods and medicines are always more easily assimilated in liquid form. It is no surprise then that the liquid essence should often be the most effective way of transferring particular forms of energy into the body.

Why flowers?

All life derives from the light of the sun. Plants which grow in the sun can be thought of as uniquely sensitive to the balance between that source of primary energy and the gravitational and other forces of the earth. Although all parts of many plants can be used in medicine, the flower – the sexual part of the plant, the shortest lived and most sensitive to the light – contains the greatest concentration of essential energy.

How are the remedies prepared?

The prepared flowers are usually placed in water in a clear glass vessel in sunlight. This is the most natural method since the sun is used to release its own stored energy. For a very few flowers, and some other parts of plants, a 'boiling method' is used but, unless absolutely necessary, this is felt to be less satisfactory and can easily destroy the essential energy unless very carefully managed. In order to improve the keeping quality, the essences are usually made up with alcohol or some other preservative; a few drops of the original essence are added to a quantity of brandy or vodka to make up the 'stock' essence. This is the form in which the essences are usually sold. For those who cannot tolerate alcohol, a pure aqueous stock can be made, but this makes storage difficult, so the alcoholic versions are the more common. The use of other preservatives such as glycerine is attracting interest but is not usual commercial practice at the moment. More details are given in the chapters on the various remedies.

How are the remedies prescribed?

Flower essences can be prescribed in a number of ways. The traditional way used by Dr Bach and his followers is simply to talk to the patient, matching the remedy to their state of mind as revealed in the interview. It is also possible to prescribe by various forms of dowsing, muscle testing or guided meditation. These approaches and the various pros and cons are discussed together with the different groups of remedies.

How are the remedies taken?

A number of drops of the stock essence are added to water, or to a mix of brandy and water, to make up a treatment bottle. The remedy can be taken direct from the treatment bottle or further diluted by placing a few drops in a glass of water. In an emergency, if it is not practicable to dilute, drops of the stock remedy can be taken neat. The number of dilutions does not appear to make any difference to the effectiveness of the remedy. Higher dilutions are preferable for those who dislike the taste or are sensitive to the effects of alcohol. In warm weather a remedy bottle made with pure water is liable to go off and should be kept refrigerated and checked regularly. If a treatment bottle is to be kept for a long time it is advisable to dilute in pure alcohol. An alternative approach which is gaining favour is to dilute with a quantity of glycerine added to water. This is a good compromise for the alcohol-sensitive and gives a much better level of preservation than pure water, although less good than alcohol. The precise dosage regimes vary slightly and are discussed with the individual group of remedies.

How do the remedies work?

The action of the remedies is most visible on the emotional level. In any condition of ill health, we know that we often 'feel better' before there is measurable improvement in the symptoms. The vibration of the body has been changed in the right direction and the physical effects will follow since the physical substance is moulded in the pattern of our energy field. The remedies, by addressing primarily the way we *feel* as opposed to what may appear to be wrong with us, work on the level of that vibration and bring us more quickly to the turning point of feeling better from which any other healing which is necessary can follow.

Are the remedies safe?

The remedies are all entirely safe: the energies used are so subtle that they can only stimulate movements which the body, so to say, wants to make anyway, and for that reason will either act for the good or not at all. There is no question of excessive action or side effects as there could be from allopathic drugs – all the remedies do is to give a minute stimulus towards right action. If more is taken than needed it will only enhance the positive aspect of the remedy. If an inappropriate remedy is taken, it will simply not act. The Bach remedies are all made from non-poisonous flowers. Some of the other remedy series do use flowers from poisonous plants, e.g. aconite but by the time the remedy is given in its dosage form, it is so dilute that the question of direct chemical action does not arise: the few adverse reactions that occasionally occur are caused by the brandy rather than the essence!

Can the remedies help with serious physical disease, or do they just work on the mind and emotions?

Modern Western medicine approaches questions of sickness and health as problems which can be solved piecemeal, as though the whole were only the sum of the parts which 'just happened' to be there and which worked together in an altogether arbitrary fashion. Traditional natural medicine has always maintained the view that human beings can only be dealt with as a whole and that sickness must be treated in a way which has regard to the whole nature. If the flesh of the body is seen as arising directly from spirit, as *in-carnation*, it follows that diseases of the body have their origin in sickness of the spirit and that when the spirit is healed it is able to heal the body. This, however, is a subtle process which can take time, and more conventional medical care may still often be needed to support the weakened body while healing from within takes place. The use of these remedies is not and was never intended to replace responsible and enlightened medical attention, but to enable it to be more effective.

Should the remedies be used alone or can they be combined with other treatments?

Flower remedies are generally entirely compatible with all other forms of treatment. The remedies will certainly not interfere with anything else and I do not know of anything that will antidote or block their effect. In many cases it may be helpful to both the practitioner and patient to use one therapy at a time, in order to be clear as to exactly *what* is having the effect, which is difficult if many things are going on at once (the same argument can be applied to combination remedies), but with more experience this becomes less important: if the right remedy is given it will act.

It is important to consider everything which may have an effect on the overall health and particularly on problems for which treatment is being given. Many conventional drug therapies, while undoubtedly effective in terms of the specific symptoms they are designed to treat, have an undermining effect on the general vitality: if this is the case, real recovery will be an uphill task. Similarly, if a problem is being constantly aggravated by a seriously deficient diet or unsatisfactory way of life it would not be reasonable to expect more than a limited result from the use of remedies alone. One needs to think in terms of *removing obstacles* to healing, so that the *stimulus* provided by the remedies can be most effective.

How do I know that the remedies I buy are genuine?

'Bach Flower Remedies®' are supplied by the Bach Centre at Mount Vernon. The name and various details of the packaging design are stringently protected by copyright. Although they are distributed very widely in commerce, there is very little chance of a properly labelled Bach Remedies bottle containing anything else. With respect to other remedies, the best course is probably to buy direct from the makers, where this is possible, or from a reputable distributor, such as the Flower Essence Association or a local supplier of integrity. I have not heard of any difficulties arising with fake, contaminated or otherwise unsatisfactory remedies but it is probably as well to be cautious (see below).

Do the remedies need to be prescribed by a qualified practitioner?

Not necessarily. In the case of the Bach remedies, Dr Bach's clear intention was that the use of his remedies should be simple enough for anyone to be able to prescribe for themselves and their family. In most cases this is really the best option, since the development of insight which comes from thinking about the remedies and prescribing them is as valuable as the effect of the remedies themselves. As a practitioner I usually talk about the remedies with my clients, firstly to ensure that they understand and agree to follow the kinds of change I have in mind for them (!) and secondly to encourage them to develop an interest in the remedies.

How do I find a practitioner?

People who work as 'Flower Remedy Practitioners' may have training varying from a single weekend workshop in one set of remedies to a lifetime's experience and a wide range of clinical skills. Don't go by a label, look for the substance and don't be afraid to ask exactly what people do and how they learned to do it. Many people who practise in related fields (myself for instance) do not advertise themselves as flower remedy practitioners as such but use the remedies, as appropriate, in conjunction with whatever else they happen to be doing. These could include aromatherapists, Bates Method (vision education) teachers, counsellors, kinesiologists, reflexologists and others.

How can I learn more about the use of the remedies?

The 'contacts' section at the end of this book gives addresses of suppliers, most of whom run some form of training seminars or consultancy. You will also find local practitioners offering courses and workshops where you can study with others who are interested.

The 'publications' section gives a comprehensive listing of available books on the subject, with some notes for guidance. It is obviously advisable to read as widely as possible if you are thinking of using the remedies regularly.

In the end, knowledge comes from experience: read, discuss, think all you can, but above all *use* the remedies and learn from the results you obtain. Buy the remedies you feel will be most useful and start by prescribing for the situations and pictures that are immediately clear to you and you will find your understanding grows in depth and subtlety from day one. Have fun!

2

Dr Bach and the English flower remedies

The first group of flower remedies known in modern times were those discovered by Dr Edward Bach (1887–1936). Dr Bach trained in medicine and early on became a convinced homoeopath. Putting his early training in pathology to good use he specialised for a time in research into *nosodes* – products of disease used as remedies. A particular group of these remedies, from diseased bowel tissue, are still known as the 'Bach nosodes'. Throughout his life he was a profoundly religious man – he took up medicine very much from a vocation to heal – and although convinced of the soundness of homoeopathy, he found the complexity of homoeopathic prescribing, to say nothing of the rather unsavoury materials with which he found himself working, rather depressing. He also felt the wish for a method of healing that was simple enough for the layman to use and that came directly from the light, so to speak, rather than having to be mined out of the darkness of byproducts of disease.

By way of relief from his work in London, he often took

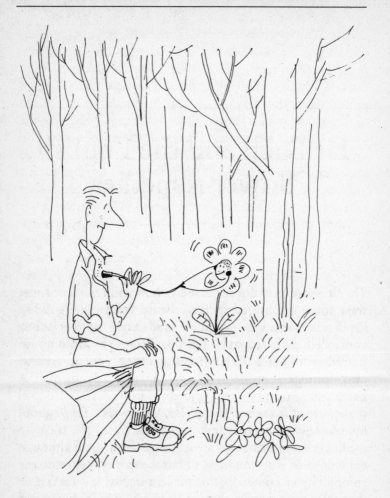

holidays in the country. Over the years, both before and after he finally quit his London practice, he spent a great deal of time in Wales and in Norfolk, where he especially enjoyed long walks in the woods and fields, alone, or latterly with his friend and assistant Nora Weeks. He began to find that in these wanderings he was intuitively drawn to

certain plants which he associated with particular emotions. Later, more dramatically, he began to experience 'out
of the blue' strange and unpleasant emotions: driven out of
doors to find relief in fresh air and exercise, he was then
astonished to find that on his walk he would find, or be led
to, a particular plant or tree and that simply being in the
presence of this plant would relieve his disturbed state. He
became convinced that these experiences had not come
about by chance, but that they were an answer to his
prayers: the feelings he had experienced and the plants that
relieved him were the keys to a new way of healing.

When the remedies reached 38 in number the experiences ceased and he concluded that his work was complete.
The 38 remedies relate to carefully delineated emotional
states which between them, according to Dr Bach, cover
the entire spectrum of human emotion and therefore form
a complete healing system to which, like the Book of
Revelation, nothing should be added nor from it taken
away. He laid great emphasis on the need for clarity and
simplicity and he is said to have specifically predicted and
warned against those who would create confusion by
attempting to improve on his work. This of course leads to
the continuing controversy in relation to the 'new' remedies, which will be discussed further on.

Dr Bach established a healing centre in a small house at
Mount Vernon in Oxfordshire where many of the plants
used in the remedies could either be grown in the garden or
were available in the wild nearby. This was obviously
important since in order to capture the *essence* of a plant
the preparation should always be made with the flowers in
as fresh a condition as possible.

Dr Bach died at a relatively young age not long after the
completion of his work. Cynics might ask why, in the
words of the title of his first book, he could not 'heal

himself' and prolong his own life? This is to fall into the common error of supposing that the point of healing is to prevent death. If, like Dr Bach, we regard this present life as only an episode and death as only a passing from one state to another, it is clear that there is no need to stay once the work one came to do is complete. After Dr Bach's death, the work of making the remedies was carried on at Mount Vernon by curators. Victor Bullen and Nora Weeks, who kept the centre for many years, had been close personal friends of Dr Bach. They regarded themselves very much as the trustees of Dr Bach's legacy and saw their rôle as the preservation of that legacy for future generations.

Victor and Nora were succeeded by Nickie Murray who continued to run the centre in the same spirit and with great success. She was assisted for a time by Judy Howard and John Ramsell who later became joint custodians, and also by Julian Barnard who now makes remedies to Dr Bach's directions under the trade name of 'Healing Herbs'.

Since nothing stands still, any activity must develop or die, and the recent history of the flower remedies shows that this can be done in different ways. The Bach Centre has naturally worked very hard to preserve the integrity and uniqueness of Dr Bach's work and also to promote it throughout the world. In the process the scale of manu-facture and the extent of the financial transactions involved have grown to an extent that Dr Bach might have found surprising. Naturally, running a business on such a scale has involved the occasional legal action to defend trade marks and copyrights, and also various attempts to control production of, and information concerning, the remedies. The business is now actually owned by Nelson's pharmacy and no doubt the additional support will enable further growth and development without compromising the qual-ity of the remedies. In this book are described the results of work by others who have chosen development by broadening the number and kind of remedies available. This is a controversial matter: the 'Bach purist' will stand by the letter of the doctor's statement that no more were needed, while those who are finding new remedies would say that the fact that they are being discovered shows the need at this time.

Julian and Martine Barnard who run Healing Herbs have chosen the path of development in depth rather than breadth. They have chosen neither to explore additional essences, nor to work at expanding the availability of the remedies but to return to the spirit of Dr Bach's work in the sense of listening to the plants themselves and also preparing the remedies exactly as Dr Bach did in the early days. They are quite happy to explore new sources for their flowers, provided that they *feel* right and this point illustrates neatly the dilemma faced by all concerned with 'maintaining a tradition'. For instance, there is an obvious and easy merit in suggesting that flowers should be taken from the original site, and if possible the same plants that Dr Bach used. But in this world, the site may now be beside a motorway or underneath a shopping mall: if the original tree is there at all it may be a decrepit, mutilated shadow of the fine young specimen that Dr Bach knew: so does one choose the form of the tradition or try to rediscover its spirit? This is a question that must be faced constantly by any who follow in the footsteps of great men, and one that must be answered by each one for himself alone.

We are always given choice: not only, as Dr Bach says, so that we can discern truth from falsehood, but also in order that we may find the path which is right for us. In that spirit, within the following pages, I have collected information on as many of the 'new remedies' as possible, without passing any judgment on their respective merits, or of other people's work or opinions: but it is right that, before all else, we should consider more closely the nature and use of the wonderful remedies which were discovered through Dr Bach's gift, and which he gave freely to the world.

3

The 38 remedies of Dr Bach

The Bach remedies are obviously the best known and most readily available flower essences: they are also the most fully described and tested, so they make the obvious starting point for anyone interested in learning to prescribe. Once the principles of the Bach system are understood, the other groups of remedies can be considered with their various differences.

The publications section of this book lists all the Bach Centre publications and a number of other books, all of which are invaluable for the would-be prescriber. Absolutely essential is the (free) descriptive leaflet which lists the remedies with brief 'keynote' descriptions. My own descriptions of the remedies given in this chapter are based on experience and may vary in detail or emphasis from those found elsewhere. I have attempted, above all, to create mental pictures which are vivid rather than technically definitive as it is with the most obvious cases that one can start prescribing with confidence and learn rapidly just how the remedies work in practice.

Agrimony Agrimonia eupatoria

Agrimony hides trouble behind a brave face. What kind of trouble? It doesn't matter, such a person's catch-phrase will always be – 'I'm fine'. Up to a point this may be admirable: there are perhaps enough people in the world anxious to share their troubles (see Heather), so that an Agrimony type's anxiety not to burden others may be very welcome. The trouble is, it doesn't stop there: the sick Agrimony may completely refuse to acknowledge to themselves that there is a problem, deeply suppressing their grief so that it grows in the dark and leads to deep pathologies.

Aptly, this first remedy shows the power of the Bach system and way of prescribing almost better than any other. The very general way of prescribing means that one does not need to dig deeply into protected areas: the fact that they are protected in a certain way says it all. The patient who may just barely be able to acknowledge a slight unease without wanting to be too frank about the details is likely to find traditional flower therapy more acceptable than approaches which would be more invasive (e.g. muscle testing) or require more detailed information (e.g. homoeopathy).

When Agrimony is successfully prescribed, it may be that the problem will dissolve without any need to disclose what it was all about, or equally that the patient may 'open up' and be able to work in ways that were previously unavailable. Either way, Agrimony often brings help to those who, because of their willingness to hide their suffering, might otherwise get no help at all.

Aspen Populus tremula

The *Aspen* tree is sensitive to the point that it trembles visibly in a breeze so slight that it cannot be felt on the skin. Warning of what cannot yet be seen, it illustrates the old *doctrine of signatures* (the plant visibly resembles the organ or the condition which it will heal). Aspen is fearful or at least anxious – of what, who knows? A nameless dread, a sense that some awful calamity is about to befall but no idea of what or why. Among other things, this suggests Aspen as a good remedy for agoraphobics and others prone to suffer from apparently causeless panic attacks. It might also be appropriate for children's fears e.g. of the dark, of being alone, in the sense that there is generally no clearly defined idea of *what* is likely to come out of the dark, etc. (If there is a more defined idea, consider Mimulus.) These conditions give a great deal of trouble to medical practitioners, who like to see the reasons for people's experiences, and who are likely to dismiss them as 'unreal' if they cannot: hence, they will usually resort to all-purpose tranquillisers which control the feeling without addressing the cause. Although the cause may not be apparent, one obviously exists for anything that happens and Aspen will find and remove it without the need for it to be named.

Beech Fagus sylvatica

The Beech character is described as 'critical and intolerant of others'. The important point to note, which differentiates Beech from the other remedies, is that Beech (in the pure form) does not have anything better to offer. The old boarding school stories always featured such a character, who would avoid getting involved in any activity but would always be present on the sidelines to jeer and scoff at the earnest souls who tried to achieve in whatever way. Sometimes this character would go in for active malevolence, in which case we would think of Holly (see below). This would be far too much like hard work for Beech as the character is not only negative in the extreme, but also essentially passive. Beech is the 'permanent opposition' present in every organisation's committee, who is always extremely good at damning the ideas and efforts of others while never deigning to offer a contribution of their own. This contrasts with Vine who may be pretty scathing in criticism, but only as a prelude to inviting you to move over and see how it should be done (and will pretty often be right).

Centaury *Centaurium umbellatum*

The Centaury character has been described as a 'human doormat'. It may well be that a Centaury type will attract

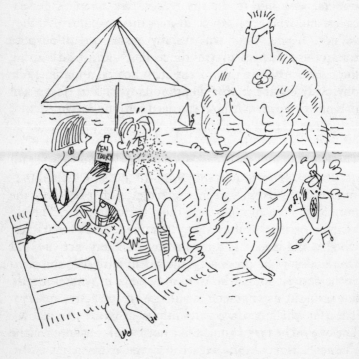

CENTAURY TYPE

partners who will be in need of a dose of Vine (see below) or something stronger.

Centaury children are bullied at school; Centaury adults are bullied by their partners; Centaury workers are bullied by their bosses; and they never complain but accept it as their lot. There is a basic lack of self-esteem which allows them not only to allow, but somehow to need, this regular abuse which does neither themselves nor their abusers any good.

This needs to be distinguished very carefully from the positive aspects of a willingness to accept discipline, to be helpful to others, and so on. One of the main difficulties with Centaury people is that they are often reluctant to seek help because what is happening to them, although unpleasant, seems part of the natural order of things. They will say, 'I don't mind doing twice as much work as anyone else in the office – I like to be helpful' and, 'Of course I don't like my husband shouting at me if his shirt isn't ironed quite right, but he works so hard and he does need to look his best so I try to understand and I don't mind really'. Centaury helps this willingness to serve to find a more positive manifestation.

Cerato Ceratostigma willmottiana

Cerato personifies one of the great pests of the world: the person who always wants advice and will never act on it. A Cerato with a headache will, typically, ring round all his friends for advice and collect telephone numbers of their osteopaths, homoeopaths, acupuncturists, Alexander teachers, herbalists and what have you. The next step will be to call all these people to discuss whether they may be able to help. This will involve not only exhaustive discussion of every detail to make clear that this is no ordinary headache, nor like any ever known in the history of humanity, but also discussion of all the opinions offered by everyone else spoken to so far ('The osteopath thought it might be a displaced vertebra – do you think that's likely?') and any ideas gathered from the numerous books he has read on the subject. Eventually, one of these unfortunates will receive the dubious honour of a visit, will go through the whole rigmarole again, give the best advice they can and make another appointment. The appointment will very likely be cancelled ('Well I was talking to my friend and he told me about this wonderful man he sees and I thought I should give him a try') or if kept will be a waste of time ('I started to take the pills you gave me but then I felt a bit funny and I wasn't sure if it was the pills or not but I thought I'd better stop and then I had to see my acu-puncturist anyway...').

This applies not only to health matters: I once attempted to teach such a person to play the piano and have frequently regretted getting involved with acquaintances who asked advice on purchases of boats, bicycles, com-puters – it really doesn't matter. The point is that the full-blooded Cerato is so anxious to do the best and only the best, that he ends up doing nothing at all, and expends a lot of his own and others' energy in the process. This can happen to all of us on occasion, surrounded as we are with endless choice and conflicting information, but if health is to be maintained at some point we say 'enough!', make a decision for good or ill and move on to something else.

A good Cerato prescription, then, will have the effect of unblocking the decision-making process, enabling us to sift information confidently in order to arrive at a balanced decision and then *carry it through*. Since the remedies also act to strengthen the positive side, it will also be useful for anyone who may not show the Cerato symptoms, but feels bogged down in decision making because of 'information overload'.

Cherry Plum *Prunus cerasifera*

Cherry Plum is for states of *violent rage* to the point of not knowing what one is doing. It is normally thought of as an acute remedy – it is hard to imagine the Cherry Plum condition as a permanent one – but the Cherry Plum type certainly exists in a state of pent-up anger which surfaces whenever it finds an outlet, through drink or some mild provocation. The Cherry Plum victim will find excuses for his (usually his, though sometimes her) behaviour: in poverty, in stress – it will often even be blamed on something called love – but many people who suffer far more never give way to these states. Part of being human is to remember that we have choice and can take responsibility, and Cherry Plum helps jog that vital memory. In some parts of the world, Cherry Plum in the drinking water would no doubt reduce the misery of battered wives and save the lives of tortured babies. Perhaps in combination with Holly, it could reduce the tendency to start and prolong pointless and bitter wars. Begin, charitably, at home next time you have an urge to smash a plate. (If you are too late, try Rescue Remedy, for yourself and those around you!)

Chestnut Bud *Aesculus hippocastanum (green buds)*

'Some people just never learn!' Chestnut Bud will help them in great things as in small. In spring every junior school nature table has its display of 'sticky buds' from the horse chestnut tree. Chestnut Bud can be an important remedy in childhood for those who get *stuck* on a task and seem to lack the imagination to find another way. Patrick Macdonald, teaching us the Alexander Technique, would say, 'If at first you don't succeed, do not try the same thing again' and was right as usual. Chestnut Bud is for those who are always trying the same thing and never able to see why it doesn't work. Later in life this can apply on a deeper level to emotional patterns and fixations: people who go through the same ritual patterns with a succession of partners, every time thinking that things will be different and every time with the same outcome. Even with great insight and the help of skilled therapists, these patterns, acquired early in life, can be dreadfully hard to change and Chestnut Bud may make it just that little bit easier.

Chicory *Cichorium intybus*

Chicory is a remedy for mothers-in-law and maiden aunts: not real ones of course, just those cartoon characters of people with a sharp tongue and gimlet eye who are always ready to give the benefit of their long and rich experience of life to any relation over whom they can claim some kind of authority, when the only aspect of life of which they have real experience is *manipulation through guilt*. There is a kind of parent who will not allow their children to grow up. This can take the form of keeping them at home, unmarried until past marrying age, or 'helping' with the grandchildren in a way that amounts to taking over since (in Granny's mind) the child parent is so obviously helpless that it would otherwise be a clear case for the social services. There are husbands and wives who treat their spouses like children, stifling them with a possessive 'love' which will hardly allow them out of sight. There is also a tendency in children at a certain age to try very hard to dominate their parents. The unpleasant and insidious aspect of the Chicory character, which sets it clearly apart from the other remedies, is the naked emotional blackmail which is used to keep control. 'If you love me', 'I can't live without you', 'It doesn't seem very much to ask, after all I *am* your mother and I don't suppose I'll be here to trouble you much longer' are all drawn from the Chicory phrasebook.

None of this is nice, but it has to be said. At the bottom of all this unfortunate behaviour is, of course, real fear and real need. People do need each other and do fear loneliness, but trying to bind your loved one in chains of guilt is no better a solution than handcuffing them to the bed. Love, if it is to be worth anything, needs to be free.

Chicory, then, if well chosen as a remedy, has the quality on the one hand of strengthening the individual so as to reduce the emotional dependency that underlies all the problem behaviour and on the other of promoting emotional honesty so that real needs can be openly expressed and lovingly met. Buy some today!

Clematis Clematis vitalba

This is not the big blue thing growing up the front of the house, but the little one with insignificant white flowers found in every hedgerow (in our part of the world at least).

Clematis is a dreamer. Clematis children can be recognised by passive faces (often round and 'mooney') and vacant eyes (frequently covered with spectacles – they often become short-sighted because they do not 'connect' with the outside world). As the saying goes: 'Sometimes I sits and thinks and sometimes I just sits' – Clematis just sits.

When Clematis is correctly prescribed to a child, the transformative effect on the young person's personality, outlook, behaviour and educational prospects needs to be seen to be believed. It is possible to see, quite literally, the eyes and mind click into focus. I would regard it as one of the most important type remedies in children, especially as the Clematis type of dysfunction seems to be one of the more common low-level side effects of vaccination.

Crab Apple Malus sylvestris

Crab Apple is described as the cleanser. On the physical

level this suggests affinity with all sorts of eruptions and skin diseases, from acne to psoriasis, and diseases needing a lot of purging, such as forms of influenza with heavy sweats. On the emotional level it relates to anything that gives rise to the feeling of being unclean or 'messed up' inside. It figures strongly in relation to sexual problems ranging from a general feeling of confusion about the whole thing, to hurt and anger that may be felt in an unsatisfactory relationship, to the feelings of soiling, revulsion and self-loathing that are commonly experienced following sexual assault. Eating disorders, reflecting as they do a dissatisfaction with one's appearance or nature and which also have a strongly sexual connotation, would also suggest this remedy. Some of the 'new' remedies deal with these problems more directly and perhaps precisely, but Crab Apple, like all the Bach remedies, addresses the feeling without needing to go into details of the cause and so can help even where there are personal or cultural taboos against discussing intimate issues explicitly. This would have been especially important perhaps in the England of Dr Bach's day. It would be wrong, however, to think of Crab Apple as an exclusively sexual remedy – feelings of self-hatred can have many causes. Quiet souls who are provoked into an outburst of anger, or house-proud people who suffer fire or flood may well experience the Crab Apple state with great intensity.

The positive side of Crab Apple is clearly self acceptance: acceptance of one's physical form with all its blemishes; acceptance of one's emotional nature with all its inadequacies; acceptance of one's personal history. In Carlos Castaneda's *The teachings of Don Juan* the nagual Don Juan speaks of the need to erase personal history through acceptance in order to become free to act through our beings instead of being trapped within them. This is a considerable task for most people, but one which the judicious use of Crab Apple can make a little easier.

Elm *Ulmus procera*

This remedy and the next two form a closely related group, and are concerned with the ability to carry through a task once chosen. Often, when climbing a mountain, the lie of the ground creates a false horizon, giving the impression that the top is very near. Ascending the ridge, you realise that the goal is much further away than you thought and suddenly your legs feel very tired and you want to sit down and cry! At this point you have to remember that the view, daunting as it is, actually shows how far you have come, that a realistic view of the situation is necessary to work out how to cover the rest of the ground, and that progress will be best made one step at a time, as it has been before. This is a very exact metaphor for the Elm 'problem' and its solution.

Elm has generally reached a certain level of success, through a degree of application, but has further to go. Suddenly, the scale of the task, the risks and uncertainties, become magnified and it all seems daunting and unattainable. In short, there is a loss of nerve or at least a crisis of confidence. The point is that there is no rational basis for this feeling: things may actually be going very smoothly and complete success may only require a 'steady as she goes' outlook, but the sense of proportion has been lost and it all seems too much, leading to depression and exhaustion.

Successfully applied, the remedy restores confidence and proportion, enabling things to be carried to their successful outcome.

Gentian Gentiana amarella

Gentian is usually described as doubting and despondent. How is this distinguished from the loss of confidence associated with Elm? By the *reason* for the despondency. Elm is despondent because the task seems too great for one's powers. Gentian by contrast feels that perhaps the task was not worth undertaking anyway, that one should have been doing something different all along and maybe it would be better to give up and change course, if it is not too late. If Elm relates to the condition usually described as 'burnout', Gentian connects very strongly to the mid-life crisis, when all that had seemed worthwhile before is called into question. If continuing on the path is the right approach, the application of Gentian will strengthen and speed the decision to carry on. If not, the need for change will become clearer so that the mind can concentrate on the practicalities.

Gorse Ulex europaeus

There's really no point in writing about this remedy, no point in writing the book, come to that – no one will buy it and if they do they won't read it, and even if they get that far they won't take any notice. Well, suppose they did, they probably wouldn't be able to get the remedies anyway because the shops would be closed or they'd forget and buy the wrong ones or they simply wouldn't work – I don't know: *What's the use?*

Yes, Gorse is for those days when you feel it's really not worth getting out of bed. On a longer-term basis, it is an important remedy for chronic invalids who despair of ever getting better. Many forms of treatment may have been tried and none has succeeded and there is a disinclination to explore further – easier just to give up and wait for the end. A number of seriously disabling diseases present this picture very strongly: one may say that it is natural to feel despair in the face of a disease which has no cure, but it is equally true that no disease will find a cure unless it is sought.

In trying to escape the grip of the malaise, the Gorse patient may invest very high expectations in a proposed course of treatment. It is easy to be fooled by the expressions of confidence and enthusiasm into missing the Gorse characteristic, but it will often be betrayed by the manner, contradicting what is said, and confirmed by the speed with which the enthusiasm evaporates if there is not an instant miracle cure. For that reason, if the Gorse picture is suspected from the history or general manner, even if not clearly presented, it is probably worth adding Gorse into the cocktail as a precaution – otherwise the patient may give up treatment before there is a chance of a result.

Heather *Calluna vulgaris*

Heather can often be prescribed with certainty more quickly than any other remedy: unfortunately, the consultations with Heather patients tend to take longer than any others because a Heather type simply has to tell you all about it, whatever 'it' is. A real Heather type, the classic saloon bar bore (male or female), will insist on absolutely monopolising the attention. The least pleasant characteristic is the habit of 'buttonholing' the victim – backing them into a corner and talking very close to the face. (In homoeopathy, *Lachesis* has the same unpleasant tendencies.) Even an attempt to avert the gaze may be taken as a sign of lack of interest, leading to renewed insistence. This may also be experienced with children, perhaps slightly backward or insecure in some way, who make incessant and unreasonable demands on a teacher or anyone else who happens to be around, and who display unusual

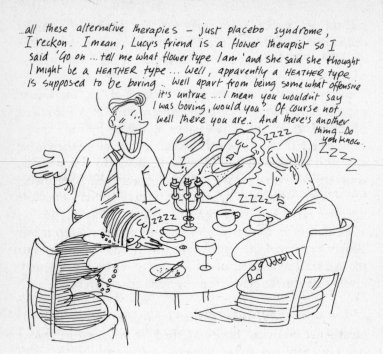

insensitivity and lack of awareness towards others. Practitioners will also be familiar with Heather as a demanding patient who is constantly ringing up to discuss their complaints and never satisfied with a quick word. In this case the medium is the message: any symptoms that are being talked about are far less important than the way the telling is done. If that sounds callous, you must bear in mind that the true Heather tends to resist cure because it is so fascinating to talk about their complaints that taking them away would spoil the fun. Therefore, whatever is wrong, if the Heather mind-set is present, it is not possible to work on anything else until that is removed. Practitioners sometimes debate the ethics of telling patients which remedies they are being given and in general there are good arguments on both sides. Generally, in using flower remedies, I prefer to think of myself as more of a teacher than practitioner, discussing the use and purpose of the remedies fully with the intention of developing the client's insight and self-reliance. The existence of the Heather personality sorely tests this plan because there is no nice way of telling anybody just why you want to give them this remedy, and no way of stopping them reading it up once you tell them the name. Although they like talking about themselves, Heather types are curiously lacking in self-awareness and are also generally short on sense of humour, and clumsy attempts to prescribe Heather are a good way of losing clients before you have had a chance to help them.

If this all sounds horribly damning, I should say that most people, me included, go through Heather phases of various degrees of severity from time to time, most likely when our enthusiasm for a particular subject causes us to fail to notice the glazed expressions and loud snores coming from our unwilling audience. Catch yourself doing that more than once and think of using Heather as an acute remedy before it becomes a habit.

Heather can be confused with Cerato. To distinguish between them, Cerato will tell you what everyone else thinks and seek your opinion on all of it (and will listen most respectfully and gratefully). Heather is much more concerned with his or her own opinions and is a very poor listener.

The positive side of Heather is seen as a much truer insight into the self, and through that a great willingness to help and sensitivity to the needs of others. Poachers turn gamekeepers and reformed Heathers often make excellent counsellors.

Holly *Ilex aquifolium*

Holly *hates* someone or something. In truth there is only one kind of hate: that directed against the self, but it expresses itself against an outside object. We tell ourselves that we hate others because they do (or are) evil, but in truth we hate them for showing us the evil in ourselves. You doubt? Look at the crowd baying for the blood of small boys who have killed another.When hate is directed violently outwards in this way, it may be confused with the Cherry Plum condition: the main difference is the focusing on an object. (The Cherry Plum rage is against the world in general and those who get hurt are innocent bystanders, or more often the nearest and dearest – those most available, anyway.) Equally, though, the Holly hatred can be kept inside, feeding on bitterness and growing in darkness.

Honeysuckle *Lonicera caprifolium*

Honeysuckle is for nostalgia, dwelling in the past, for the feeling that the future has nothing to offer and consequently for a lack of interest in the present. This can apply to the longing for a lost love, or simply for the feeling that things were better in the old days. It could be an important remedy in relation to some visual problems e.g. short sight, where there is a basis in emotional distress relating to a loss. It also bears on many of the problems of old age, where an advanced form of the honeysuckle condition can lead to a sort of living death. The positive aspect of honeysuckle is a lively enjoyment of the present which is supported by a strong sense of continuity with the past.

Hornbeam *Carpinus betulus*

Does every morning feel like Monday morning? The kind of day when you have a whole list of things to do but somehow it seems absolutely necessary to have another cup of tea and then just a little look at the paper or at the TV? Eventually arriving at your desk, you feel an urgent need to have another look through last week's post before sorting the paperclips into their different colours, then finally you begin work on that urgent report when, good heavens, it's time for coffee – 'Well I'd better have some, it might wake me up, why do I always feel so tired?'

Cheer up – you are not alone: without the aid of copious quantities of Hornbeam I should never have completed this book.

Impatiens Impatiens gladulifera

Impatiens – the 'Busy Lizzie' of a million garden tubs – is so called because of its rapid and profuse growth. In a striking illustration of the doctrine of signatures, it applies very literally to people of an impatient nature. Impatiens is a great remedy for young children – on journeys (think of travelling without the chorus of 'Are we nearly there?') or to calm the excitement of the run up to birthdays and Christmas. It can also be thought of for children (or adults) who fail to learn because they lack staying power: the type who start a project full of enthusiasm but lose interest before it is half complete, or those who constantly change jobs because they can never find satisfaction. Impatiens children have 'ants in their pants' while their grown-up counterparts often appear to have equally itchy feet. Impatiens can also be short-tempered – the type who does not suffer fools (who appear to make up most of the rest of the population).

Impatiens needs to be carefully distinguished from Vervain. The general manner, in particular the feeling of rushing around and wasting energy, may be quite similar, but the point is that Vervain will usually get things done, possibly exhausting himself and everyone else in the process but getting there nonetheless. Impatiens far too often just doesn't get there at all. The timely prescription of the remedy allows all that energy and quickness of mind to be put to better use.

Larch Larix decidua

The Larch picture resembles that of Elm but describes a more permanent state. Whereas Elm suffers a temporary loss of confidence within an overall context of competence and success, Larch suffers more from what used to be described as an 'inferiority complex' and is entirely certain of being no good for anything. The remedy can be a very important aid in building confidence, initiative and the willingness to take risks that is essential for a fulfilled life.

Mimulus Mimulus guttatus

Fear is possibly the most negative of all emotions. It not only paralyses the will, preventing a situation from being changed, but it also attracts the thing that is feared so that the prophecy based on fear is always self-fulfilling. The importance of Mimulus as a remedy is that if we can stop creating problems for ourselves in that way, we can make the energy available to address real problems that need our attention. Mimulus contrasts with Aspen in that the Mimulus fear is always of something definite. It may be of an impending event, of a disease, of old age or dying, it matters not: whenever someone says 'I am afraid of ...', Mimulus is the first remedy to use.

Fear is so potent and so ingrained in many of us that it is almost certainly advisable to combine the application of Mimulus with suitable counselling or therapy aimed at changing the attitude to the object of the fear. Perhaps the commonest and strongest is the fear of death. What is the point of being afraid of dying when it is the inevitable end point of all life? It cannot be prevented (although much medical practice seems to encourage the illusion that it could, if only more money were spent) so surely we should spend our energy on living well, however we conceive it? Yet so many people, having been told that they suffer from a 'fatal' disease, immediately stop living, afraid to do anything, to experience anything, in case it brings their end a minute nearer. Before their diagnosis they would never have given the matter a moment's thought, yet what is the real difference in their situation? This is the reality and the absurdity of fear and yet it is hard to cast it out of our hearts, even if our minds are convinced of the truth of what I have written. Mimulus helps us not just to accept this important message with our intellect, but to truly take it to heart and to live more freely and more fully as a result.

Mustard Sinapis arvensis

This is not the stuff you put on your steak! Rather it is the aromatic woodlander known in some parts as 'Charlock'. In contrast to Mimulus, Mustard relates to a condition with *no known cause*: a despondent gloom which descends, as it were, out of a clear blue sky and hovers over the head of someone who has no reason to be anything but happy and content. Before prescribing Mustard one should take care to eliminate the usual suspects: the Gentian despondency of uncertainty, the Elm loss of courage, the Hornbeam lassitude and procrastination, the Centaury down-troddenness and many others.

Mustard only fits the case if there is no reason at all. This means that, while it may be suggested fairly often at first sight, when cases are analysed more deeply some other remedy is actually required. If the true Mustard case is a little rare, it is very graphic when encountered and for that condition there is not only no other remedy but probably no other form of therapy that will help: it is truly essential.

Oak *Quercus robur*

Oak is an unusual remedy which describes a particular type in a particular moment. It is for strong brave people who are on the point of being overwhelmed. This needs to be carefully contrasted with the Elm crisis of confidence. Elm imagines that it is all too much and is tempted to give up, although everything is fine – the problem is a loss of sense of proportion. Oak imagines that he can go on forever, when in fact his strength is ebbing and the crisis is all too real. This therapeutic contrast between the two quintessentially English trees is mirrored in their form and behaviour: the towering graceful Elm has always been notoriously whimsical, given to dropping branches at random and letting itself be killed off by beetles; while the shorter, more prosaic Oak hangs on to its last breath even after being struck by lightning.

Olive *Olea europaea*

In the Mediterranean world, the olive tree was almost regarded as the 'tree of life'. We would expect its essence to be a little special and so it is. Olive describes a state of *absolute* exhaustion. I emphasise this because it is one of the remedies (Sweet Chestnut is another) that should only be used when absolutely necessary. If you take Olive when just a bit off colour (perhaps instead of Hornbeam) it will probably do nothing at all. Taken when you feel about to drop to bits, however, it will work miracles (but not if it has already been taken prematurely – be warned). The exhaustion may be mental, spiritual or physical, and frequently all three. It follows that Olive should almost certainly not be used as a 'type' remedy, nor generally in chronics. If there is a genuine chronic state of total exhaustion, other remedies will most likely have the key to the cause. Dr Bach is not known to have travelled in the Mediterranean and it must be assumed that his encounter with the Olive tree took place in England – possibly at Kew. It has been suggested that plants from the native locations would make a better remedy than those from hothouse specimens.

Pine Pinus sylvestris

Pine is for feelings of unjustified guilt. Guilt is never a healthy emotion: if something has been done wrong, acknowledge it, make whatever amends are possible, make a point of not doing it again and forget it. If it continues to trouble you, consider it as an ordinary obsession and think of the suitable remedies. The Pine victim, usually female, persists in feeling guilty for things that are not only not their fault but often none of their business. It is one of the classic 'mother's remedies', along with Chicory, Cerato and Red Chestnut. I once asked someone: 'If anything goes wrong in your house, whose fault is it?' Without hesitation she replied 'Mine!' Her automatic response to any situation, whether of her making or not was 'Sorry'. After a week of Pine, her life was her own again.

Red Chestnut Aesculus carnea

The flower of the Red Horse Chestnut is another 'mother's remedy', with the key of 'excessive care for others'. This is for the wife who sits trembling every evening certain that her husband will have had an accident on the way home, the father who lies awake every night until his eighteen-year-old daughter is home and in bed, the grandmother who worries herself to death over her grandson, certain that he will be abducted if he walks two yards alone, that he will die of pneumonia if he gets his feet wet, and so on.

The picture can relate very closely to that of Chicory, since the 'care' can become a potent tool of manipulation and one that is hard to fight without appearing selfish and ungrateful. Extreme cases of the Red Chestnut condition appear in highly dysfunctional families, including those identified by R.D. Laing as tending to schizophrenia. Even in lesser forms it destroys the lives of both the 'carer' and the victims of their care.

Successful prescription of the remedy helps develop perspective in individuals and better, freer relationships between them.

Rock Rose Helianthemum nummularium

Rock Rose is one of the component remedies in the Rescue Remedy. It expresses extreme fear to the extent of panic and terror. Mimulus is afraid of something known, Aspen of something unknown. With Rock Rose the source of the fear is immaterial: for whatever reason, the patient will be absolutely terrified, probably physically affected and quite incapable of facing the object of fear. This can relate either to a real source of fear, a memory of a terrible accident perhaps, or something purely imaginary, giving rise to nightmares. Its action overlaps with the homoeopathic Aconite and Belladonna, both of which encompass stark terror, but can be freely given, regardless of physical symptoms, etc. and with far less concern about the precise dosage.

Rock Water potentised spring water

Rock Water is unique among the flower remedies in not being made from flowers, but from the water of a spring found close to Mount Vernon. Rock Water people are hard on themselves. They have fixed ideas about right and wrong, and work very hard to set the world a good

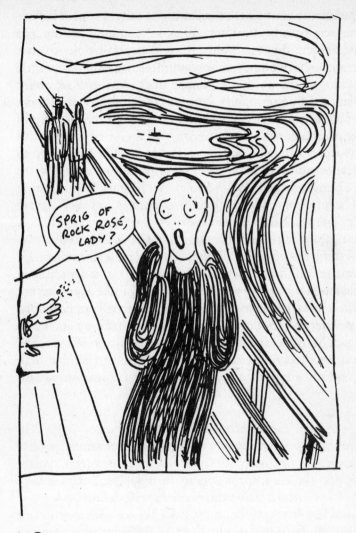

ROCK ROSE EXPRESSES EXTREME FEAR
... TO THE EXTENT OF PANIC AND TERROR

example. Whereas Beech will criticise other people's behaviour very openly and Vine will make strenuous attempts to make others do as he wants, Rock Water will look on other people's shortcomings in sorrowful silence and, with a little shaking of the head and pursing of the lips, will set about doing the thing properly. Personal relationships with these people are very difficult because, although they say nothing, they are very good at giving off an air of disapproval and their own behaviour is so constrained by their need to demonstrate perfection that they appear aloof and cold.

The aloofness of Water Violet (q.v.) comes from wanting to be left alone: Water Violet lives a quiet and very private life. The real Rock Water type lives much more in public so that the example of virtue should not be overlooked.

I think the point here is that it is all very well having high standards and setting a good example, but it won't have much effect on anyone unless they either like you or think of you as someone to emulate. The cause will not be helped if you acquire the reputation for being a stuck-up crackpot, which is often the fate of a negative Rock Water. The positive effect of the remedy is to allow one to see that high standards are perfectly compatible with common humanity.

Scleranthus Scleranthus annuus

Scleranthus is the remedy of *choice*. Other remedies have the quality of uncertainty, but Scleranthus relates specifically to the choice that has to be made between (usually two) options that are in themselves well defined. Someone in a Scleranthus state of mind does not seek advice and will probably be found alone, deep in thought, or abstracted and preoccupied in company while he turns the problem over (the classic theatrical Scleranthus is Shakespeare's Hamlet). It is a condition which affects highly principled people, perhaps unclear as to the course of duty or torn between conflicting loyalties, or perhaps slightly less principled people, wrestling with a bad conscience.

Scleranthus needs to be clearly distinguished from Cerato. This can easily be done on two points: Cerato is dealing with numerous options (the Scleranthus problem is more clear-cut) and will share the difficulty with all and sundry (Scleranthus, as we have said, will keep it to himself).

Scleranthus successfully prescribed leads to quick and clear decision making, with great savings of energy and time as a result.

Star of Bethlehem *Ornithogalum umbellatum*

Star of Bethlehem is another of the constituents of the Rescue Remedy. Its action very closely resembles that of that other great healer, the homoeopathic Arnica characterised by physical or mental shock. It applies equally whether someone has just been involved in a car crash, heard that their child has been killed, or witnessed an accident. All these things will lead to that condition of being suddenly detached from the body, of not quite knowing where one is or what day it is; not being able to take in what has happened. It has been suggested that what actually happens in these instances is that the bond between soul and body is temporarily weakened – one is literally knocked out of oneself – and that the remedy acts to reunite the two as firmly and speedily as possible.

Sweet Chestnut *Castanea sativa*

Sweet Chestnut is another of the life-saving remedies: it is for absolute despair. As with Olive, don't use this lightly or prematurely but when it feels that the world, in a personal sense, has truly come to an end, when one is simply drowning in grief (and this happens at least once in a lifetime to all except the unlucky few) Sweet Chestnut is your only man. Grief is such a profoundly important emotion that many people are extremely reluctant to use remedies of any kind while grieving as it seems that relieving the pain will somehow rob them of something. This may be accurate in relation to orthodox therapy, since tranquillisers and anti-depressants relieve the pain by actually blocking off the ability to feel. It is important to understand that the flower remedy works in a completely different way – far from blocking off the feeling, it unblocks the source of emotion, enabling it to move freely until it finds its own resolution. It is wrong and does a great disservice to describe a vibrational essence of this kind as a 'herbal tranquilliser' as I have heard more than once. When the body is free to respond fully to grief, or any other source of pain, the end result is always cleansing and strengthening.

Vervain Verbena officinalis

Vervain is a basic remedy for all northern Europeans and anyone else brought up in the grip of the Protestant work ethic – the idea that to do anything well requires effort. A Vervain type is often a classic over-achiever, always on the go, diligent, conscientious and successful. The main problem seems to be an inability to enjoy the fruits of those labours, to recognise that there is a time to stop and relax. This leads to problems of physical tension and fatigue, and also puts a great strain on intimate and family relationships, leading to unhappiness in that area.

In many other cases, Vervains are triers who under-achieve because they regard effort and the appearance of making effort as important in themselves, whether or not they produce anything. This can lead to all kinds of learning and performance difficulties, since the mind only functions really well when relaxed. Besides the emotional problems mentioned above, this can lead to tremendous frustration and eventually great bitterness (Willow) because they feel it unjust that their honest efforts are not better rewarded.

In these times of great awareness of stress, many people invest time and effort in stress management courses, yoga and meditation classes and even electronic devices to help them relax. For a Vervain type, none of these will work because, at a deep level, he does not feel that being relaxed is right and does not understand that it would be more productive. The remedy will not only help directly, but it will also make all these other activities much more useful. The positive Vervain state is well balanced, applying the necessary effort to do the job rather than straining away for the sake of it.

Vine Vitis vinifera

The basic polarity of Vine is leadership or tyranny. This is an important remedy because in a highly socialised society we need leaders and invest them with a great deal of authority to rule us and act on our behalf. The history of the Twentieth Century is largely the story of societies ruined by investing in the wrong leaders, or the leaders being ruined by being unprepared to handle power. Why do so many of the 'great men' of history turn out on close inspection to be hysterical, cowardly bullies? Part of the answer is that others are prepared to let them get their own way, but another part is their own failure to know themselves and to direct their ambitions properly.

The aggressive and even delinquent tendencies seen in many young boys and men are often the negative side of strong leaders. Such boys are often encouraged into outdoor and physical pursuits in order to 'channel their energies into something constructive'. The problem is that causing delinquent bullies to become very fit and offering them a rich experience of life merely creates very fit, experienced bullies. In order to really rechannel the energies, something has to cause a fundamental change of heart and Vine is potentially that something.

In the business world, until recently, willingness to negotiate with inferiors was seen as a sign of weakness and a manager would be regarded as effective in proportion to the loudness of his voice. Fortunately, that culture is rapidly changing, but many people still in that particular rut will need Vine as well as Walnut (see below).

In a positive state, the Vine type exerts leadership skills for the service of others, rather than wielding power for its own sake. Negotiation and concern for those led takes the place of bullying. The level of willing co-operation which results guarantees greater success in any enterprise, whether it be a football team or a nation. As in the case of Olive, Vine was probably encountered by Dr Bach in captivity. The early preparations were certainly made from cultivated varieties and it has been suggested that wild stocks from native locations may be more effective. Healing Herbs currently prepare their Vine essence from a wild source in Greece and report very good results.

Walnut Juglans regia

Walnut is a remedy of changes. In a sense all remedies act on this point since it can be truly said that life is a process of constant change and disease is the result of resistance to change. Walnut is usually thought of particularly in relation to major life changes such as moving house, bereavement, separation, etc., and where these things can be anticipated it is worthwhile to take the remedy as part of a process of preparation for the event, perhaps over weeks or even months, and to continue through until the change has been assimilated. More subtly, one can perhaps identify as a Walnut 'type' someone who is unusually or unhealthily resistant to *any* change in their life. This could apply both to those for whom the social mores of their forefathers are the only possible options for good, and to those who, in our youth- and beauty-obsessed culture are dismayed to the point of self-destruction by the prospect of ageing.

When Walnut is successfully prescribed the changes which must come can be seen as more or less interesting features of the journey in life, rather than as obstructions or its end.

Water Violet Hottonia palustris

Water Violet is a modest retiring sort of flower and the characteristic of Water Violet types is that they are very quiet and keep to themselves. They sometimes acquire the reputation of being unsociable or 'stuck up' but it is really more a question of being self-sufficient and not really needing constant communication with others. In itself this trait is both rather appealing and probably quite healthy (at least, you'd think so after spending an hour with Heather).

With a remedy like this it is important to remember that, although the remedies are prescribed on emotional pictures, the main intention is not necessarily to *change* the person's character. In some cases the behaviour and character may not alter at all, but the remedy, suitable to the type, will help whatever ailments they may have. In other cases, the character will be altered only in subtle ways that reinforce and emphasise the positive aspects. Only where there is a distinct lack of balance will a big change in the actual behaviour appear, but when it does there will almost certainly be big improvements in other areas.

A Water Violet personality can be entirely psycho-
logically healthy but still be helped by the remedy in
physical ailments which may stem from a degree of
rigidity.

The unhealthy Water Violet condition can in some ways
resemble Agrimony or Rock Water in their less extreme
forms. The difference from Agrimony is that there is no
great grief hidden, nor an effort made to conceal it, just a
sense of *reserve*. Water Violet compares to Rock Water
rather as a Quaker to a Presbyterian. There may appear to
be a lack of ability to feel things fully, almost an emotional
numbness. Such people may appear painfully shy or be
made definitely ill by contact with others. In that case the
positive effect of the remedy will be to open out the
personality gently so that the quality of quietness will be
seen to stem from genuine inner tranquillity rather than
from self-denial and rigid 'holding in'.

White Chestnut Aesculus hippocastanum
White Chestnut is very much a remedy for the modern age.
It is the remedy for a condition in which thoughts control
the mind rather than the mind controlling thought. Cir-
cling, repetitive thoughts that go nowhere take a number of
forms. There may be a single obsessive preoccupation
which completely blocks other thought; or there may be a
mass of conflicting and competing ideas and demands
which squabble among themselves like angry starlings
without ever reaching a resolution; then again, there can be
a generalised state of over-excitement brought on by a
stimulating play, concert or book. In all these cases normal
thought processes are drowned out by the noise.

The main effect is an inability to be *present*: the
preoccupying thoughts may be of the past (White Chestnut
is often an alternative for Honeysuckle) or dominated by

plans, dreams and speculations concerning the future (in this case White Chestnut may be the correct remedy for a case that would at first sight suggest Clematis). The White Chestnut condition can have a similar feeling and outward appearance to that of Scleranthus: the difference being that Scleranthus is struggling to find the answer while White Chestnut is still working out the question. It is also related to Cerato, but Cerato will project the confusion and incessant questioning out onto others, while White Chestnut will normally keep it to himself.

White Chestnut can be sometimes mistaken for Clematis: intense preoccupation with the interior dialogue can give a similarly vacant impression to the outsider, but careful enquiry will reveal the internal activity. White Chestnut looks blank because there is too much going on inside, while Clematis looks blank because there is nothing going on.

White Chestnut can be extraordinarily effective in the acute situation: it is a great remedy for insomnia after parties, concerts, etc. The chronic condition is more difficult because obsessive thought is strongly habit forming. In the same way that someone accustomed to being surrounded by noise of traffic and radios and TVs all the time can be disconcerted by the quiet of the countryside, so the person whose mind is usually filled with noise and chatter may be quite unprepared for the silence of a clear mind and will often go to some lengths to fill it up again. No remedy can be used against the will of the user, conscious or unconscious and repeated abuse will desensitise to the point where the remedy will no longer act. If this is the case, an extended course of White Chestnut should be accompanied by suitable work on the part of the patient to consciously change the habits of using the mind.

Wild Oat Bromus racemosus

One proverbially 'sows the wild oats' before settling down to a regular life and the Wild Oat remedy is for those who are finding that settling down difficult. This seems to me to be another remedy of great importance at the present time, because, for young people especially, the question 'What shall I do with my life?' has never been more pressing.

As little as 50 years ago, most people, in Britain at least, could have their career pattern predetermined by the end of

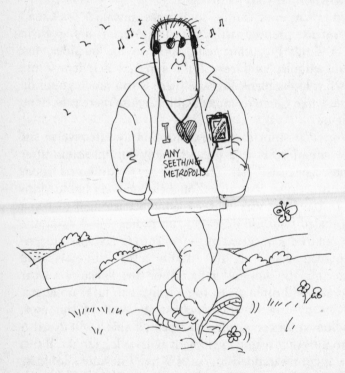

...SOMEONE SURROUNDED BY NOISE OF TRAFFIC
AND RADIOS AND TV'S ALL THE TIME CAN BE
DISCONCERTED BY THE QUIET OF THE COUNTRYSIDE...

their first year in school, if not as soon as they were born. Son would follow father down the mine or into the doctor's surgery; daughters would marry suitably, or work within a range of acceptable occupations and so on. Rapid social and industrial change, accelerated by two world wars has completely changed that picture. Whole occupations have been swept away, children no longer live in the same towns or cities that their parents grew up in and those parents all too often have no jobs for the children to follow them into.

Although the demise of secure employment for life with large paternalistic corporations and collectively bargained fair wages is unsettling, it is very much in tune with the essential spirit of the present age which is the increasing need and willingness to take responsibility for ourselves and to make our own decisions, to meet our own needs. 'What to do with my life' is the most important decision we shall ever take: how, out of the present morass of possibilities to find something that will continue to inspire and challenge us, and that will make a valuable contribution to society. The use of Wild Oat shows very clearly that taking a remedy is no substitute for action. It can only help if you are prepared to get out and do something (if that is a problem, think of Hornbeam), but it will make it all a lot easier.

Wild Rose Rosa canina

The keynote of Wild Rose is apathy. Acceptance of that which cannot be changed may be a virtue, but Wild Rose is fatalistic to a fault. Whatever happens in life, health, partnerships, work, they will accept with a shrug and say 'Well there's nothing I can do, is there?'

This can be infuriating, but instead of picking them up and shaking them, try a few drops of Wild Rose.

Willow Salix vitellina

The favourite phrase of a Willow type is 'It's not fair!' If someone else has a better job, better health, lower golf handicap, Willow will be there to say 'What's *he* done to deserve such luck?' Well maybe he didn't irritate providence by moaning all the time, for a start. Willow is the proverbial character who 'Wouldn't be happy if he was happy'. Even if things do look up, he'll be the last to admit it. Most therapists of any kind know this character:

'How's the back?' (He has been immobilised with pain for ten years.)

'Oh, all right I suppose, but my foot's been hurting all week.'

When this sort of thing drives you to the limit of exasperation, don't shout or commit violence – give them Willow instead.

How is Willow differentiated from Beech? Beech's negativity is very much directed outwards at others: Beech does not criticise out of envy, far from it! He would not want to be in the shoes of those poor fools (as he regards those he criticises) for anything. Willow's feeling is far more personal: he very precisely wants to be in the other person's shoes (and suit and carrying his briefcase and sitting behind his desk and living in his house) and the lack of these things causes him great unhappiness.

The transformation brought about by Willow can be quite miraculous. This negative, moaning, wet blanket starts to see the funny side of things – even of his own misfortunes. He will probably start to learn from experience instead of complaining about it. He might even see that other people have some good points. Well – it's got to be worth a try!

Rescue Remedy® composite (Cherry Plum, Clematis, Impatiens, Rock Rose, Star of Bethlehem)

Every household in the world should have a bottle of Rescue Remedy®. Many people have been entirely converted to the use of the Bach remedies without reading a single book, solely by seeing the effects of this wonderful essence.

Although it is a compound of remedies that are available singly in the set, the Rescue Remedy® is considered as a distinct and single remedy in its own right. It is designed for use in emergency situations and of course it is right that at such times one can do without even a slight hesitation over which is the right remedy. Basically, if the situation is such that *something* needs to be given *right away*, Rescue Remedy® is always the right one. When the emergency is over and there is time to reflect, other single remedies may play an important part in restoring balance.

It is hard to think of anyone attempting to bring up children without Rescue Remedy®. Children fall downstairs, wake up with nightmares, have fights and tantrums, suffer illnesses which are at best uncomfortable and can be frightening if only because they do not understand what is happening. Rescue Remedy® in all these situations does a lot to restore family harmony. In our family, it has been so much used in temper tantrums that the children will ask for it in mid-howl. Clever little ones: in the heat of our adult rows it is all too easily forgotten.

My son Edwin (aged eight at the time) attended a canoeing course at which basic first aid and resuscitation was taught. He returned home in disbelief: 'Do you know, they had never *heard* of Rescue Remedy®?!' He was quite right: in situations of shock and exposure, Rescue Remedy® can be a life saver (together with the correct first-aid procedures, of course). If the patient is unconscious, so that it would be unwise to give anything by mouth, simply wetting the lips with a drop of the remedy (stock or dilute) is all that is needed for the patient to get the benefit of the remedy. (This also works well with uncooperative children.)

Mental shock, from whatever cause, can be a killer: separation, bereavement, house fire, witnessing (as opposed to being involved in) a road accident, all do great damage to the nervous system and can weaken the bonds between the subtle energy bodies and the physical. Rescue Remedy® is invaluable in all these cases (especially when people say they are all right and don't need anything).

The range of situations where the Rescue Remedy® applies really underlines Dr Bach's commitment to simplicity. Each one of the situations outlined above could involve one of a number of homoeopathic remedies in one of a range of potencies. Arguably, the correct one of these would act more powerfully on the individual case – assuming that they were all available together with someone with the knowledge and time to sort out which one to use. The beauty of Rescue Remedy® is that it will work pretty well in all the circumstances suggested – and many others – and can be used without any hesitation. Buy three bottles, keep one in the kitchen, one in the car and one in your handbag or briefcase. And use it.

4

Working with the flower remedies

The information given in this chapter applies to the Bach remedies and to most flower and other essences generally. Any significant variations in the way of working with other groups are described together with the remedies in later chapters.

BEGINNING TO PRESCRIBE

Having formed general pictures of the individual Bach remedies, we can look in a little more detail at the process of prescribing. The only teacher is experience. Reading will give you information, but only prescribing remedies and seeing the results of your prescribing will teach you their correct use. Rescue Remedy® shows the power of the flowers to the most sceptical: many people have used it for years without bothering about or even knowing of the other remedies, but, wonderful healer that it is, Rescue Remedy® is still only a part of the system and learning the use of even a few more remedies can open up whole new worlds.

PRESCRIBING FOR YOURSELF
AND OTHERS

Prescribing for yourself is not always easy but can be very instructive. We do not see ourselves entirely as others do, nonetheless most of us have some insight into our states of mind and are able to verbalise our feelings. Perhaps in reading through some descriptions of remedies some particular phrase will strike a chord of recognition: that's me, that's just how I feel! All right, take the stuff and see what it does for you. There is of course the possibility that *all* the remedies will seem to be absolutely essential! If this is the case, aim to find one or two that seem more essential than the rest but if you really can't, take likely candidates one at a time and see how you feel!

Prescribing for others is for many people a most daunting prospect: the responsibility – 'what if I get it wrong?' Relax: it is actually quite hard to go wrong and even if you do no harm will result. In any case, rather than rushing to give remedies to all and sundry, you will do best to begin by not actually prescribing at all but by thinking about the remedy pictures and using them as a lens through which to focus on the behaviour of those around you. Just by reading and observing, you will begin to recognise the patterns of individual and interactive behaviour that relate to each remedy. You will then begin to identify situations where an offer of help might be appropriate (and those where it most definitely will not!) and soon will have made your first successful prescription. Charity begins at home and your first prescriptions will almost certainly be for yourself, your family and immediate friends. Remember that willing consent is essential, however, and beware of your own enthusiasm. I know to my cost how easy it is to lose friends if the 'terrible urge to do good' is so strong that you become a proselytising zealot or simply a bore (if you catch yourself falling in that direction, consider Vine and Heather).

THE INTERVIEW

Dr Bach's method of prescribing was based exclusively on listening to the patient talking. Essentially, the method is to identify from the patient's speech key feelings or ideas which correspond to the different remedies. The 'pictures' of the remedies were, of course, very clearly engraved in Dr Bach's mind: the rest of us have some learning to do. This is not so hard, however. Given that there are only 38 remedies and that the only symptoms to be considered are mental and emotional, it is quite feasible to keep the characteristics of the whole set in one's head. (Compare that with homoeopathy where it is necessary to learn at least several hundred remedies – out of possibly thousands – and with symptoms for every part of the body and the simplicity of the Bach system does look rather appealing.) In any case, it is not necessary nor advisable to try to learn all the remedies by heart before attempting to prescribe. Listen to what people say, ponder it while glancing down the key list of remedies, and read more deeply on any that seem to apply.

KEYNOTES

Although the remedies have many facets, most of them, as you will have seen in the previous chapter, can be asso-ciated with a particular key phrase or 'keynotes' which sums up the essential idea. It is amusing as well as amazing how often these phrases turn up in the conversation of patients, quite unconscious that they are speaking the very words set down by Dr Bach in his books. Gorse patients really do say 'What's the use?', while 'It's just not fair' is a surefire pointer to Willow. It is perfectly correct to say that one cannot prescribe reliably from the keynotes alone: they are intended primarily as an 'aide memoire' to be used in conjunction with a full study of the descriptions. However, once a remedy is known and understood, the keynote serves as a 'memory peg' which is sufficient to bring the whole picture to mind.

TYPES AND OCCASIONS

It could be said that, whereas remedies are generally prescribed on the way you feel, the *type remedy* is prescribed on the way other people feel about you. Describing a person as the *type* of a particular remedy suggests behaviour that is so habitual that we would say 'the person is *like that*'. Of course, no one really *is* 'like that', they just *act* 'like that', but if they do it often enough the behaviour becomes seen as part of the person.

Most of remedies correspond recognisably to 'types': Beech, Centaury, Heather, Vine, to name a few at random, all have strong *type* associations. Equally, they can all occur on an *occasional* basis in people who do not conform to that type, or any other – Beech is appropriate for all of us when we give in to the impulse to destructive criticism, Centaury when we allow ourselves to be dominated by bullies, Vine when our enthusiasms turn us into that bully, Heather when those same enthusiasms make us buttonholing bores.

A type remedy can be taken on a long-term basis as part of a concerted attempt to create change – it is not a good idea to just keep taking remedies if you are determined to stay the same – or, more conservatively, as a first resort whenever one is out of sorts and no other remedy suggests itself.

A few remedies do not really occur as types: Walnut and Star of Bethlehem, for instance, relate to acute rather than chronic conditions which do not persist long enough for a set type character to take hold. It is not generally recommended to use Rescue Remedy® as a type, or for chronic cases, but I have done so on occasions, mainly in cases where a person seems to be very much affected by childhood injuries and where nothing else seems to apply. For long term use it is better, however, to identify the single remedies that apply, if at all possible.

ONE OR MANY?

Remedies can be prescribed singly, in sequence or in combination. Combining remedies has many possibilities: any number within reason can be mixed together in a 'cocktail' and all the ingredients should act on the appropriate elements in the person. There is, as in anything, a right and a wrong way to approach this.

The great thing *not* to do is to abuse the licence to prescribe multiple remedies by the 'each-way bet'. There is a temptation to give all the remedies suggested by a particular condition, say, Gorse, Gentian and Larch (all remedies which express, say, a lack of confidence) at once because in a particular case you may not be sure which one is needed. This is obviously wrong, because you know perfectly well that two out of the three will not be needed and it is only mental laziness that prevents you from making the attempt to differentiate clearly between them. Moreover, by working in that way, you make sure that you will never become any clearer.

The legitimate use of multiple prescribing is in the case

where the problem covers a number of well-defined remedies. An abused woman, for instance, may need Centaury (she allows exploitation) but also Pine (she feels it is all her fault, that she deserves it) and Agrimony (she covers up her distress to all her friends and family). In a case like this (entirely hypothetical) one, it is fairly clear that all these areas, which are distinct although part of the same problem, need to be covered and that the cocktail can be seen almost as creating a new, specific remedy for the situation.

There is a great deal to be said, however, for prescribing single remedies whenever possible, for a number of reasons which have especial force in the early stages of learning:

- Seeing the single remedy act gives more definite feedback: there is no confusion as to *which* remedy is having the effect.
- The attempt to prescribe a single remedy encourages one to *prioritise*: out of a number of issues in the case, which is the most important right now?

In relation to the first example given above (wrong prescribing), it is obvious that if after due deliberation you are still not sure of the right remedy, it is better to give the 'shortlist candidates' one at a time. The inappropriate ones will not act and when the correct one does, rereading the descriptions and comparing them with the facts of the case will help you to see through your confusion.

In the second kind of case, although this way of working is perfectly sound, I would still ideally prefer to give remedies one at a time (although possibly in quick succession). This is partly because I feel it is an excellent discipline for the prescriber to disentangle and sort the various strands of the problem and, more importantly, because it enables one to get into the case in a more detailed way. Healing a person can be compared (very loosely!) to restoring a painting. Removing the first layer of grime on your old master may reveal something quite unexpected which will change your whole attitude to the project. Similarly, giving *only* the remedy which seems most essential, the 'top layer' remedy, may change the picture entirely so that the next and subsequent prescriptions may be quite different from those you would have given at the first interview. In acute situations I have often found it best to sit round the table with all the remedies to hand and give different ones as indicated by the changes of feeling that occur. Ten remedies in an hour would not be unusual, and this way of working can be very effective.

It is largely a question of practicality. It is obviously far easier to change remedies frequently if you are regularly in touch, e.g. in the family situation, than if you only see someone at six-week intervals. A great deal also depends on how involved the patient is with the use of the remedies. With someone who is sufficiently interested and aware, rather than give a dosage bottle with a cocktail, I would encourage them to buy stocks of all the indicated remedies and ask them to use their own judgement as to which one to take and when. Combine this kind of approach with fairly detailed reporting and both patient and practitioner can learn tremendous amounts. On the other hand, with someone who does not really want to know much about the therapy, but just wants to be given help (which is their prerogative) the cocktail may well be the best approach.

STORAGE, PREPARATION AND DOSAGE

The remedies should be kept in reasonably cool, dark conditions, away from any strong aromas, and preferably with the bottles not physically in contact. The storage boxes provided by suppliers have dividers to make this easy. Although the normal stock tinctures are well preserved, it is a good idea to avoid contamination: for example, if you take drops direct from the stock bottle, do not let the dropper touch the mouth.

Remedies for intensive use can be simply made up with a few drops of stock added to a glass of water, which may be used at intervals for as long as it keeps fresh. For use over a longer period it is more convenient and economical to make up a treatment bottle – most pharmacies sell plain dropper bottles. The exact dilution is not important. The standard for most remedies is two drops in any reasonable quantity of water (but with the Australian remedies the dose is seven drops). Drops from the treatment bottle can be taken direct on the tongue or further diluted in a glass of water which can be kept handy.

WHAT IS IN THE BOTTLE?

One question which can be debated endlessly is whether, or to what extent, it is good for people to prescribe for themselves, or to know what they are taking (or why). Among homoeopaths and flower remedy practitioners there is a definite divide between those who name remedies and those who do not.

In favour of having someone else prescribe and not being told, it can be argued that patients can be too ready to read up the descriptions and then:

- Persuade themselves that the remedy is working when

it is not and distort consultations by describing the way they believe they ought to be feeling rather than the way they actually are.

- Take offence and possibly stop treatment if the description they read contains something that they regard as untrue, or even a slur on their character.
- Start prescribing for themselves (and stop paying the practitioner!).

In favour of full disclosure it can be argued that it is a more adult way of going on to make the interaction between prescriber and patient one of informed co-operation rather than dependency:

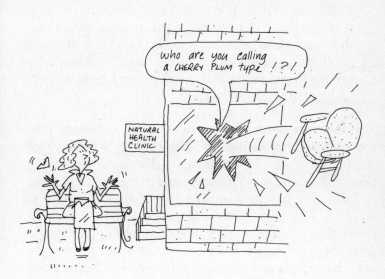

- The first argument against has some force: most patients will at some point 'read themselves into' the remedies, but after a while the novelty wears off and genuine insight replaces self-delusion. It is certainly true that on first reading of the descriptions, most of us feel that we need all of them and that an experienced prescriber will be much more easily able to discriminate what is needed.
- The second point is more problematic – it is hard to find a nice way of telling someone why you want them to take Heather and Beech (on the other hand, is it ethical to base a prescription on an opinion about someone that you would not express to their face?)
- As to the third point, in a sense, the whole idea is to stop going to practitioners and take charge of yourself. It is legitimate to be anxious that patients who think they know more than they do may do themselves no good: it is not legitimate (in my view) to deliberately mystify the process as a way of keeping paying customers tied to the apron strings.

This dilemma is one that has to be solved individually by everyone who prescribes for anyone else, whether professionally or not. My approach is always to discuss my prescribing as fully as I feel able, and to encourage patients to learn and use the remedies for themselves as far as possible. That said, with some people, who are less self aware than others, I may feel it is more appropriate just to prescribe – for a time at least. The aim of the prescribing over that time is to bring them into a state of balance and to aid the growth of their awareness so that it becomes ever more possible to include them fully in the process.

SUPPORTING TREATMENTS

In many cases, the use of the flower remedies will come about in the course of doing some other work. For instance, in my work as a Bates Method vision educator I frequently use flowers to assist with the emotional side of visual difficulties. Equally, someone consulting a prescriber of flower remedies may well ask if there is anything else they can do that will help besides 'taking the drops'. As suggested in the introduction, although it is perfectly possible to use the flower remedies alone, it is often helpful where possible to combine their use with other healing modalities.

Generally, although there may be exceptions, if you are under treatment of any form which is having a beneficial effect, it is a good idea to continue it alongside the use of the chosen remedies. The remedy cannot interfere or be interfered with, but it can make it easier to accept the benefits of therapy. It is not so much the question, for example, whether or not you undergo surgery. It may be that your condition improves so as to make the surgery unnecessary, but it may also be that the effect of the remedies will be to remove fear and apprehension from the process, giving you a more comfortable stay in hospital and less likelihood of following complications. The following ideas may also be useful:

Affirmations

An affirmation is something that you say to yourself repeatedly in order to change your habit of thought. Very often, it is helpful to use an affirmation allied to the intended effect of the remedy you are taking. Why is this necessary – should the remedy not do the job anyway? In many cases it will, but sometimes it needs a little help, or at least the withdrawal of opposition. If you have been in a chronically negative condition for a very long time, there is likely to be a very well-established mental habit which resists change. This often proves to be the case with patients who show benefit when they first take a remedy but then relapse, and find that after enough repetitions of this cycle the remedy no longer helps. Invariably in these cases, what has happened is that the patient has decided, more or less unconsciously, that the altered state of mind, although it is noticeably healthier, feels unfamiliar and therefore wrong and that to be in the former, unhealthy state feels more 'normal' and therefore 'right'. The force of the mental habit has overcome the force of the remedy. This demonstrates an important point about the supremacy of human free will – if we choose to make ourselves sick there is no power in heaven or earth that can prevent us, and if we are to be healthy, we must deliberately choose to become so! If there is a conflict between conscious and unconscious intentions, it is likely that the prevailing habit will win out, and so the main use of affirmation is to reveal and resolve these unconscious conflicts.

Some would say that this demonstrates that it is 'merely faith' and not the remedy that acts – the 'placebo effect'. Apart from the fact that, if so this 'mere faith' must be pretty good stuff and something we could all do with a little more of, this is entirely wrong: how do I know? Because the remedies act on children who are too young to have any ideas at all and who have been completely unresponsive to any form of comfort; because they act on adults who are completely unaware that they are taking anything, or that there is anything wrong with them; because they act demonstrably on plants and animals; because the wrong remedy will not act; and, indeed, because even the right remedy will sometimes fail to act, even though the patient may have the utmost confidence and faith; and so on. Affirmation is not so much a matter of talking yourself into beliefs as talking yourself out of them; it is not a matter of creating anything by force or effort, but simply removing the greatest obstacle to healing – the negative creation of our own minds.

Movement

Flower remedies in general and the Bach remedies in particular deal with emotions above all and emotion is largely a matter of movement. E-motion implies an outward movement of feeling from within and most emotional difficulties can be thought of in terms of that movement being stuck in some way. In history, many attempts to find emotional balance have taken the form of movement. All kinds of dance are involved either with the expression of emotion or with the attempt to release feeling through a state of ecstasy (ex-stasis).

Physical exercise, from the brisk walk to hard labour or yet more drastic forms, has been considered a cure all for every kind of emotional ill. Wilhelm Reich, who trained in psycho-analysis with Freud, later named the concept of 'armouring' – the process by which emotion is stifled by making the body rigid, i.e. by preventing movement – and a great deal of Reichian therapy involves re-enabling the body to feel through vigorous and sometimes violent movement exercises. Other movement techniques attempt a more subtle integration of body, mind and feeling, for instance yoga, the *eurythmy* developed by Rudolph Steiner and the self-healing work of Meir Schneider. Underlying any successful movement work is, of course, an increased awareness of how the body is moving and this is the province of the Alexander Technique.

A number of the flower remedies have the characteristic of stiffness and will help to create the capacity for freer movement. Just as with mental habits, however, it can be definitely helpful to work consciously and deliberately with the willingness to move more freely and to experience feeling through movement.

Massage

Massage, of all types, is another way to encourage life and movement into the body. It also addresses very deeply the way we feel about and react to other human beings. Inevitably, those who might be said to be in the greatest

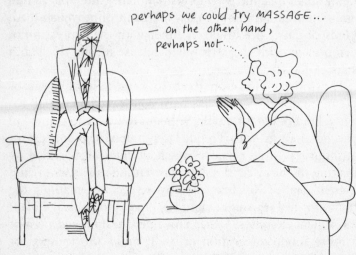

perhaps we could try MASSAGE...
— on the other hand,
perhaps not......

...THOSE WHO MIGHT BE SAID TO BE IN THE GREATEST NEED OF TOUCH, THE MOST STIFFENED AND WITHDRAWN, ARE THE LEAST LIKELY TO SEEK IT OUT OR PERMIT IT.

need of touch – the most stiffened and withdrawn – are the least likely to seek out or permit it. They will need to do other work (especially with suitable flower essences) before they are able to accept this particular benefit. For those able to accept it, physical stiffness or restriction of any kind will obviously respond to direct work on the body, but only if it is done with full consent. This is why the kinesiologist will always ask and obtain permission (of the body rather than of the patient's conscious mind) before beginning work: the rest of us just have to learn great sensitivity to any resistance.

The Russian/Israeli teacher and healer Meir Schneider has shown the effectiveness of healing 'massage' using light percussion by the fingers, rather than the conventional stroking and pulling movements. This is because the percussive touch encourages the muscle fibres to separate, as well as doing more to stimulate the circulation, whereas stroking and pressing actually maintains the coagulated state.

Subtle forms of massage, such as shia-tsu, which applies pressure to stimulate the flow of energy in the acupuncture meridians, can play a big part in releasing energy blocks in a rigid body.

Massage techniques in combination with suitable flower remedies are especially valuable to:

- Those who need movement but are in too frail a state to benefit from exercise.
- Those who lack, or are frightened of, physical contact with others.
- Those who benefit from remedies mentally but are unresponsive on the physical level.

In suggesting these additional approaches, I am not suggesting that flower therapy is inadequate or incomplete, merely emphasising the importance in undertaking any kind of healing work of an approach that is 'person-centered' rather than based on enthusiasm for our particular therapy. Flower remedies are an immensely powerful tool with a great deal of scope, but if something else is needed it should be used. The key question should always be: 'What is the matter with this person, and what is there that I, or anyone else I know of, can do about it?'

5

'New' remedies and new methods

In chapter 2 I discussed briefly some of the ethical and other questions raised concerning sources of the remedies. Different questions entirely are raised concerning the relationship between the Bach remedies and the various groups of newer remedies. The traditional position is to refuse to recognise any other remedies than the 'Bach' set, citing Dr Bach's own prohibition of 'extensions or alterations'. The book *Questions and Answers* by John Ramsell sets out the view of the Bach Centre – generally unenthusiastic – on these developments.

While this view definitely commands respect, it is beyond doubt that many of the 'new' systems are being created by people of great sincerity and goodwill, and who, if they are to be believed, are receiving guidance from spirit sources not at all dissimilar to those which guided Dr Bach. Some even assert that the spirit of Dr Bach himself is their guide! Whether one accepts this or not as 'true' is immaterial as in the end the only thing that counts is whether the remedies have their desired and intended effects. It also appears that flower essences prepared in a very similar way to the Bach remedies have been known in other cultures for centuries, in which case, from a global perspective, Dr Bach's discoveries cannot be seen as either unique or unprecedented.

My personal view is that the Bach remedies will probably meet the needs of most people in most situations and that, with sufficient thought, most conditions can be identified in terms of the Bach rubrics. However, I also think it is fair to say that there is a difference between adding to or altering the Bach system and the creation of completely new systems. Dr Bach's creation survives intact and self-contained and remains as he intended – a wonderfully simple and powerful healing tool. But that is not to say that there is no merit in systems that are more complex and require more training. These systems should, however, be regarded as separate and be judged on their own merits rather than as 'extensions' to or 'improvements' on Dr Bach's work. Dr Bach tired of the complexities of homoeopathy and wished to change his own practice but he never suggested that homoeopathy be abolished or that anyone should be prevented from practising it if they chose, nor that it was an effective and necessary therapy. Different therapeutic systems address different levels of our being and, as different individuals are most receptive on different levels, different systems are needed.

New essences for new times

It is also true that the Bach systems, although in one sense of timeless and universal value, in other ways can be seen as particularly expressive of Dr Bach's own time and place and, some would say, limited by it in some respects. While the nature of human emotion may not have changed very much over the last 50 years, the nature of its expression and the level of people's self-awareness has certainly altered.

Ian White (see chapter 7) states that the Bach remedies 'did not address areas such as sexuality, communication, learning skills, creativity and spirituality'. This may strike some as a bit sweeping since, intelligently used, the Bach remedies can do a lot of good work in these areas and it can be held as a virtue of the Bach system, especially in relation to the British temperament and most especially in the climate of the 1930s, that deep difficulties can be treated without a great deal of intimate disclosure. In different times and places where a more 'upfront' approach is generally encountered, it may be true that addressing these issues in a much more explicit and detailed way, as happens with the recent introductions from California and Australia, is more helpful. There are obviously pros and cons here; but the point is that one has a choice and can select the most appropriate way of working for the individual case.

While the Bach remedies are depicted entirely in terms of *emotional* states, felt and expressed, some of the other remedies, as will be seen, work from quite different reference points. Some relate more directly to the physical (John Ramsell, in *Questions and Answers*, suggests the term 'Liquid Herbal Remedies' for those which work in a definitely physiological way). Others claim to bypass the physical and emotional to connect directly with the more subtle spiritual aspects of life. It has been suggested that certain groups may be appropriate at particular stages in development and not others: some writers state quite plainly that one would need to be 'evolved' to a fairly high level in order to benefit from particular remedies. (This could be contrasted with Dr Bach's aim for his remedies to be useful to all humanity and their ability to work on just about anybody.) It would be helpful in a way to make some clear distinction between the different spheres of action, rather than lumping all under the term 'essences', but this is not easy since the distinctions are not clear cut.

THE PLACE OF POWER

A number of writers suggest that there is a shifting centre of energy in the world which manifests in different locations according to the needs of the time, enabling discoveries and developments to be made for the benefit of all humanity. According to this line of thought this 'power centre' was present in Britain in the 1930s – the time of Dr Bach's discoveries – and it manifested in California in the 1970s, before moving to Australia, and so on.

With new groups of remedies springing up in so many locations, it is often asked whether there is a particular affinity between the remedies of a location and people native to that place – are the California remedies best for Americans, and Bush flowers for Australians, for instance? Ian White's answer, with regard to the Australian essence, is that it is OK as long as you don't feel actively hostile to the idea of Australia, and even better if you actively like it.

The same principle can, no doubt, be applied to all the other 'national' groups including, of course, the Bach remedies. Some Australians at the present time may feel less than warm to the idea of Britain, in which case, following the same logic, the Bush essences would probably serve them better than Bach remedies.

SAME PLANT – DIFFERENT REMEDY

Here and there botanically identical or closely related plants occur in different remedy groups with rather different descriptions. This possibly needs some explanation. The plant can be thought of as a vehicle for the energies of the locations in which it grows, so that questions such as the latitude (which affects the day length and the angle of the sun's rays), the kind of soil, altitude, the hemisphere (gravitational and magnetic forces act differently in the south and north), open or shady site, time of day and year the flowers are gathered and even the other plants predominating in the particular location, may well make a difference. Dr Bach was very particular that his remedies should be made from plants from the original sites, and this has been strictly adhered to by the Bach centre, since even the identical plants from a few miles away may be quite different. It also happens that quite different plants have confusingly similar common names. For that reason, wherever possible throughout this book I have given the botanical name alongside, which should help to reduce any confusion on that score.

NON-CONVENTIONAL PRESCRIBING

Together with the new remedies there are new ways of prescribing, and another area of possible controversy is between those who regard as unauthentic any form of prescribing other than the interview in which the essence of the remedy is sought in the patient's own words, and between those who use other techniques because they find they work. As I said earlier, many of the newer remedies relate to different reference points from the emotional pictures used by the Bach set and so necessarily use different modes of prescribing. If, for instance, the description of one of the California remedies refers explicitly to a particular *chakra* or *meridian* (see pages 78–80), the diagnosis would involve some means of assessing the energy balance in that area directly. The required information in that case would simply not be available from the conventional interview.

The fact that the new remedies are more numerous and involve more complex descriptions means that it is difficult to keep all the variables in mind. It may be difficult even to choose which *system* is best to use, never mind the actual remedy. The purist might at this point say, 'Told you so – that proves Dr Bach was right', but others would say that there is no problem provided one has some appropriate means of making the selection.

DOWSING

Divining by means of a pendulum or divining rod has been used for thousands of years as a way of obtaining information not available to the conscious senses or the rational mind. How it works is still unclear but it has been sufficiently verified, particularly by the professional water finders in Australia and elsewhere, to be beyond doubt. It seems fairly clear that real energies are involved, but so subtle that the only instrument capable of detecting them is the combination of the human body and the dowsing implement. Medical dowsing can be used in a number of ways. Used over the body of a patient the pendulum may indicate areas that need attention or points where a correction needs to be applied. In selecting essences, the patient or practitioner can dowse for the single remedy, or group, most closely related to the patient's condition.

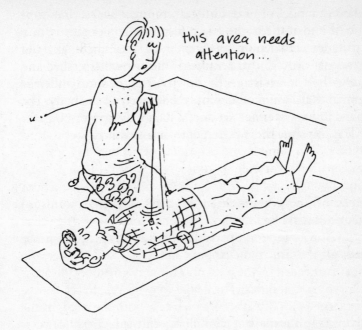

KINESIOLOGY (MUSCLE TESTING)

Muscle testing can be thought of as a more sophisticated form of dowsing by which the practitioner can obtain direct information about states of energy in the body and corrections required. The principle is that the basic tone of an individual muscle depends on the electrical activity in that part of the nervous system, which in turn reflects the activity of the brain and the system at large. Anything which stresses or 'challenges' the system will induce a weak response, while anything which relieves a challenge will induce a strong response. Various kinesiology systems use this principle in more or less complex ways, but it is possible to test for the basic response to contact with a substance very simply, using as 'indicators' the muscles of the upper arm. The patient holds the arm outstretched and is required to resist gentle downward pressure while the remedy is held in the other hand or placed on the body. The correct one will either produce a distinctly firm response or at least one markedly different from any other.

INTUITIVE DIAGNOSIS

Most of the commonly used non-traditional forms of diagnosis and prescribing depend on some degree of intuition. Some people consider themselves able to dispense with all the props and appear simply to 'see' the remedy which is needed by the patient. This may go alongside other 'clairvoyant' abilities. The healer may be able to see 'auras' or energy fields directly, in which case both the need for the remedy and its effect can be confirmed. This form of diagnosis will generally take place in a fairly conventional interview, but the practitioner will be working not so much from the words she or he hears as from what she or he 'sees' while the patient is talking.

MERIDIAN AND CHAKRA DIAGNOSIS

Oriental medicine systems describe the body not only in terms of its physical structure, but in terms of the energy structure which is the 'pattern' for the physical. Indian traditional medicine focuses on the *chakras*, or energy centres, which largely correspond to points of concentration in the parasympathetic nervous system. These can be thought of as important points of contact between the physical and energy bodies, and are certainly centres of great electrical activity. Chinese medicine refers to a system of *meridians* which are the lines along which the subtle electrical energies flow around the body, independently of the circulation or nervous system. Ill health is considered to arise from blockage or stagnation in this flow of energies and the techniques of acupuncture and acupressure are designed to remedy these imbalances by inserting needles into, or pressure on, key points. In accordance with the idea expressed earlier, that the energy body is prior to the physical, the oriental physicians maintain that changes in the energy body, which can be detected as imbalances in the chakras and meridians, indicate developing states of ill health long before physical symptoms occur, and that appropriate treatment can then rebalance the energies and so prevent the appearance of the disease which would otherwise occur in the physical. It is on this basis that Chinese doctors have traditionally been paid a retainer by their healthy patients, forfeiting their fees (or worse) if one should become sick – a vastly preferable system to one where doctors profit from continuing ill health. Several of the modern essences refer explicitly to these forms of diagnosis, and obviously, in order to make use of this information, the state of these subtle energy systems needs to be assessed.

A lot of the theory of kinesiology is based on these energy systems and the main branches include sophisticated routines for assessment and correction. More directly, the skilled practitioner can diagnose by sensing with the hands which acupoints or chakras are in need of attention. This has been scientifically validated by studies of the electrical resistance of the skin which have shown that the acupoints have far lower resistance to electrical current (i.e. allow more movement of energy) than 'normal' areas. The alterations, and the points affected, have been shown to accord with the predictions of traditional diagnosis. Traditional acupuncture treatment has also been shown to bring about normalisation. This has recently led to the development of techniques of electronic diagnosis, using an electrical probe connected to a computer to measure the resistances at various points. The computer programme then works out the pattern of any irregularities to arrive at a synoptic diagnosis, provided, of course, that the information with which it is programmed is up to the job.

OLD OR NEW?

In the end, the question of whether the new essences and different prescribing techniques are a valuable addition to our healing resources or an unhelpful aberration cannot be settled by argument, only by experience. My personal experience to date is that those I have used have certainly been effective and I am welcoming the opportunities that come my way to use others and learn more. Their existence does create complications – for those who want to get involved. Anyone who wants to keep things simple has only to leave them alone.

In the following chapters, I compare the emotional pictures of the various new essences with those of the Bach remedies in some detail. This is not to set one group up as superior to another, nor to suggest that any one essence can substitute exactly for another. My idea is simply to make clear the relationships and differences so that we can begin to see the kinds of situations where a particular remedy or group may be especially helpful. In any case, quite apart from the actual merits of the remedies, there is great value in the descriptions as tools to focus our analytical thoughts on the nature of the problems we are dealing with.

Comparing different descriptions of the same remedy and those of different but related remedies can only help to sharpen our perception of what is going on with the patient.

Together with the remedies I mention various forms of diagnosis and complementary treatment suggested as most appropriate. I do not express any opinion about any of this since the people who have done the work are in a far better position to know what they are talking about. Inevitably, as individuals, some of the remedies and the ideas expressed about healing will appeal more than others: those are the ones to use.

I have grouped the remedies roughly in order of their chronological appearance, generally treating the larger groups separately and smaller groups together, for convenience. Although some groups are better known and more popular than others at present, it would be extremely impertinent to describe any as 'more important' than others: all of them have been discovered and introduced for a reason and only time will tell which are the more significant contributions.

Some of the better established groups of essences are becoming fairly widely available in specialist shops: others are more normally obtained directly from the makers (details are in the information section pages 191–194).

6

The California essences and the Seven Herbs

ORIGINS

The California flower essences are produced and were largely developed by Richard Katz and Patricia Kaminski, who now direct the Flower Essence Society in Nevada City. As they describe it, Katz and Kaminski began their experience of flower remedies with many years of working with the Bach remedies but felt 'called' to explore the therapeutic possibilities of American native plants. The first few essences began to appear in the late 1970s and increasing interest and success led to the formation of the Flower Essence Society.

The remedies are divided into two main categories: the 'professional' kit of essences which numbers 72, and the 'research' essences of which there are over 200. The professional essences are considered to be sufficiently fully described and understood so that they can be reliably prescribed from verbal case analysis in the same way as the Bach remedies. The research essences are those which, although they have demonstrated definite potential for healing, have not been so fully described and are still undergoing evaluation. They are therefore considered more suitable for use by specialist practitioners using methods such as dowsing, muscle testing or pure intuition. Information from work of this kind and other modes of research is being collated with a view to consolidating the pictures of these remedies to the same level as the professional kit. There are 24 of the research essences which at an advanced stage of development, are included in the FES repertory and are especially drawn to the attention of practitioners with a view to arriving at definite pictures as soon as possible.

CHANNELLING

The other main source of information on these remedies is 'channelling' – the direct reception of information by a 'channel', or medium, in trance from spirit guides. Needless to say, this practice, like several aspects of the California remedies, is a little controversial, although there is, in principle, no reason to find it any more incredible than the manner by which Dr Bach apparently made his discoveries.

The channelled information is recounted in the book *Flower Essences and Vibrational Healing* by Gurudas. Here, 112 essences (the professional set and 40 others) are described in detail, the material having been channelled through Kevin Ryerson and Jon Fox. Their principal guiding spirits are named respectively as 'John' generally regarded as the apostle of the gospel, and 'Hilarion', who, it is stated, has been helping mankind with technical information of various kinds for several thousand years.

This information and the very existence of these remedies seems to many to clash head on with the claim to
uniqueness of the Bach remedies. Answers to this challenge
are offered on a number of levels (and are echoed in the
justifications offered for most of the other 'new' remedies).
As far as Katz and Kaminski are concerned, the fact that
they, in all sincerity, felt the need to go beyond Dr Bach's
work, would appear to justify breaking his ban. Gurudas
goes much further, however.

According to 'John', Dr Bach was by no means the
original discoverer of the flower remedies, but the *redis-
coverer in modern times* of knowledge that had been
commonplace in the ancient world, but lost. 'John'
describes two ancient civilisations, Lemuria and Atlantis.
The Lemurians lived in a time when the relationship
between matter and pure energy was still rather fluid:
'John' indicates that their horticulture was entirely accom-
plished through the mind and that they 'designed' and bred
plants for very specific purposes which included the further
development of the human race. The later civilisation of
Atlantis was very interested in technology and made
marvellous machines, but in taking that path lost the ability
to influence matter directly through their own faculties.
The Lemurians, living in close harmony with their surroundings were not given to sickness and the emphasis in
all their work with plants was positive development. The
Atlanteans, becoming alienated from nature, encountered
disease in the modern sense and their work with flower and
plant essences was more concerned with developing a
technology of healing which gradually turned away from
the spiritual approach of the Lemurians and towards
something more mechanistic and materially based, akin to
modern allopathic medicine. The present trend away from
this kind of approach and back to something more in

harmony with natural life forces is seen as recapitulating the Lemurian/Atlantean pattern of development in reverse.

The information provided by 'John' about the various remedies covers many facets of their history and use. As well as emotional and mental states they are related to specific aspects of physical anatomy and physiology; to the subtle anatomy (meridian system and chakras) and the relation between the physical and subtle (astral, etheric) bodies; to astrological and karmic influences; to plants, minerals and other healing influences and to the history of their development and use in Lemuria and Atlantis. This bewildering array of information is summarised in a number of useful cross-reference charts and supplemented by a vast bibliography covering all the topics raised.

PRESCRIBING THE CALIFORNIA ESSENCES

Given the large number of remedies and the complexity of the remedy pictures, it is not surprising that a number of different prescribing modalities are used with these essences. Kinesiology, pendulum dowsing and intuitive methods are all used very extensively, but it is also perfectly possible for someone who knows the remedies well to prescribe in the traditional way, from interview. The FES repertory is invaluable in this as repertorisation can quickly narrow a case down to a handful of remedies for detailed study.

THE ESSENCES

In the general scheme of things, the California essences can perhaps be thought of as forming a bridge between those remedy groups such as the Bach and Australian Bush remedies, which are very much grounded in the physical life, and those like the Alaskan and Himalayan essences, which aspire to 'higher' or, at least more esoteric things. The descriptions allude to both areas and to the connections between them, leaving it open to the individual prescriber to emphasise one or the other, or to attempt the full synthesis. Even for those who do not prescribe these remedies very often or at all, studying the literature opens the mind to a much wider perspective on how remedies work and their range of operation.

There are a number of themes that occur repeatedly, with variations, in different essences.

On the emotional level, the main themes are:

- *Sexuality* – there are many essences focused on particular aspects of sex and intimacy.
- *Social integration* – how we relate to people in groups, rather than intimately.
- *Work* – motivation, application, relationship to success, etc.
- *Life* – the relationship between the material life and the spiritual world: body, mind and spirit.
- *Growth* – maturation and ageing, child/parent, the inner child, dying.

These areas of course are not entirely separate and overlap to some extent. There are also some, mainly described by 'John', which focus particularly on various aspects of physical health and do not have marked emotional pictures.

It is beyond the scope of this small book to list all the essences, let alone discuss them fully. In any case, there is little point in duplicating the work of others, so I have mentioned only a representative selection of the more widely useful ones, mainly from the professional kit, and confined detailed discussion to those which raise particularly interesting points in themselves or in relation to other groups. For further information refer to the original sources and suppliers. For the remedies mentioned but not fully discussed, the keynotes are given to indicate the general range and to help selection of those that may be of particular interest. I would recommend that essences marked with an asterisk* should *not* be casually self-prescribed: the emotional pictures are not obvious and subtle diagnosis, by kinesiology or other means, is probably the safest and most reliable way to proceed.

I have followed the FES repertory in putting the positive key first with this group. Although all flower essences are concerned with developing positive traits, the descriptions of the Bach remedies (and the Australian Bush essences) do put a strong emphasis on the negative state to be overcome, whereas Californian essences tend to emphasise positive aspects from the outset, particularly in those whose pictures include more of the spiritual dimension.

Almond *Prunus Amygdalis**
Positive: normal growth, acceptance of maturation.
Negative: stunted growth, fear of ageing.

Aloe Vera
Positive: balance of creative forces.
Negative: 'burnout'.
This is an intensely physical remedy. The raw juice of Aloe Vera is widely considered to be a very powerful healing agent in all sorts of conditions from skin affections, to stomach ulcers, to cancer. The common theme is the failure to recover from traumatic stress which has broken the link between the physical body and the shaping force of the energy body (see page 79): hence the chronic failure of the physical body to heal and hence also the emotional picture

– which is one of giving up and being thrown into disorder. The weakening of this link is advanced as a reason why, as we age, we become more prone to scarring and distortion from injuries which in earlier life heal without a trace, and more prone to diseases such as cancer, which arise from uncontrolled growth. Where the emotional picture and the physical symptoms coincide it is recommended to use the two modalities together.

Alpine Lily Lilium Parvum
Alpine Lily is a specifically 'female' remedy which relates to positive and negative attitudes to one's body and sexuality.

Amaranthus Amaranthus Hypochondriacus*
Like Aloe Vera, this is a remedy for the extreme consequences of sustained mental and physical stress. It is indicated as being of possible use in conditions such as AIDS and schizophrenia.

Angelica Angelica Archangelica*
Another 'extreme' remedy, mainly of the nervous system, indicated for sluggish response tending to autism or schizophrenia: lack of integration, both as regards information and physical tissue – hence physical damage to nerves.

Angel's Trumpet Datura Sp
Positive: acceptance of transition.
Negative: fear of death.
The poetic common name (from its signature shape) suits wonderfully the purpose of this essence. The ability to approach death with a tranquil (as opposed to tranquillised) mind is perhaps one of the most important gifts we could ask for. (An acute state of terror as death approaches can also be helped by Aconite, in homoeopathic potency.)

Education about death is one of the most pressing needs of the present age (perhaps when we've learned to be a little more lucid about sex and birth it will become possible). Meanwhile, for those who have not developed their own resources sufficiently, such a remedy may make a vast difference to life's most important moment of transition.

*Apricot Prunus Armeniaca**
Another subtle remedy indicated for the physical manifestations of a failure to reconcile internal conflicts.

Arnica Arnica Montana
Positive: integration, feet on the ground.
Negative: disconnection, from shock.
The action of Arnica as a flower essence is identical to the mental characteristics of the homoeopathic potency.

*Avocado Persea Americana**
Positive: openness, emotional clarity.
Negative: confusion of feelings, insensitivity to touch.

*Baby Blue Eyes Nemophilia menziesii**
Positive: trust, innocence.
Negative: insecurity, defensiveness.

Banana Musa Paradisiaca
Positive: balance.
Negative: imbalances, between mind/emotion – yin/yang.
Banana is associated especially with the balance between the two sides of the brain, and also with various chemical/mineral imbalances. In relation to male sexuality, it is considered helpful in achieving a balanced attitude towards women.

Basil *Ocimum Basilicum*

Positive: integration of sexual and spiritual.

Negative: polarisation of sexual and spiritual.

Many of the modern remedies are directly and explicitly aimed at sexual healing. It could be thought that the character of this remedy could be assumed under the general rubrics of the Bach Crab Apple, but there is a good case for a more 'focused' approach.

The inability to integrate sexual urges in the context of loving relationships, or to maintain any awareness of what sex is for beyond physical gratification, is at the root of many ills. The prevalence of pornography, prostitution, rape and child abuse points to the fact that the world is teeming with lost souls, cut off from each other and from themselves. George Orwell, in *1984*, a satire on life after the Second World War, described the use of this kind of alienation as a deliberate tool of social control. It is not possible to ascribe full consciousness to the motives of many contemporary governments, but it is definitely true that our society, whatever the stated intentions of those who run it, encourages a view of sex as a furtive transaction between bodies, rather than a loving interaction between the souls dwelling in those bodies. The uselessness and the underlying hypocrisy of the standard moral and legal 'remedies' are significant. Preaching restraint, restricting display, setting age limits and putting people in prison, while using titillation as a tool – virtually the only tool – of marketing is no substitute for facing and trying to heal this alienation.

At the time I am writing this, every newspaper contains stories of scandals and crimes at all levels of society which indicate the need for this change of heart: the widespread use of this essence might bring it about sooner (see also: *Sticky Monkeyflower*).

Bells of Ireland *Malluccella Laevis*

This is another 'physical' essence, concerned with the ability of tissue to heal and regenerate and to respond beneficially to other healing energies.

Blackberry *Rubus Villosus*

Positive: decision, concrete action.
Negative: vagueness.
Blackberry is an essence for *manifestation*. Some people dream their dreams in their heads, others 'dream their dreams awake' and turn them into reality. Are you one of the first? Would you like to become one of the second? Blackberry. Now.

Black-eyed Susan *Rudbeckia Hirta**

Positive: full consciousness.
Negative: repression and avoidance of the 'dark side' of the self.

Bleeding Heart *Dicentra formosa*

Positive: unconditional love.
Negative: relationships based on fear and dependency.
The signature of the heart-shaped flower has always drawn attention to this group of plants. *Dicentra Formosa* is a small pink-flowered form, not the 'bleeding heart' of gardens, which is *Dicentra Spectabilis*, a taller and larger flowered plant with an authentic splash of blood red. No matter, this is the one that works. It operates very powerfully in relation to broken relationships – not only love affairs that have ended, but bereavements, friends who have moved away, family members who have become estranged. As an overtly emotional remedy, most of its characteristics could be covered under Bach rubrics – Walnut, Honeysuckle, possibly Chicory, would be the

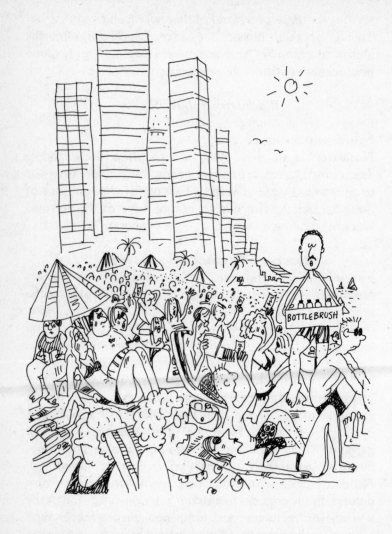

BOTTLEBRUSH (CALISTEMON VIMINALIS) ... ALSO FOR
THE STRESS OF OVERCROWDING..

starting point and others would need to be worked out individually. This essence, however, encapsulates the key idea of recentring in the self, so that although we may miss or mourn for another person, their absence does not knock us off balance.

Borage Borago officinalis

Positive: optimism, courage.
Negative: lack of confidence.
The effect of this essence is very closely related to the stimulating effect of Borage as a herb. It clearly overlaps with a number of Bach remedies – somewhere between Oak, Elm and Sweet Chestnut, depending on the degree.

Bottlebrush Callistemon Viminalis

This is a different although closely related plant from that used in the Australian Bush essence of the same name. It is a remedy for strain: the physical strain on muscle tissue brought on by over-exercise (cf homoeopathic Arnica) and also for the stress induced by overcrowding. Gurudas applies this to plants and animals: extrapolating from this, in human terms, it may well be useful in situations of tension at the community, as well as the individual, level.

Buttercup Ranunculus occidentalis

Positive: self-esteem.
Negative: low self-worth.
Buttercup deals with the sense of worth which does not depend on other people's reactions or one's position in the world. The miserable genius/millionaire and the happy pauper/idiot are not just clichés from children's stories but common characters in life. Why are so many rich and 'successful' people so unhappy? They are the people who, having inherited the whole world and lost their own soul in

the process, have profited nothing. Equally, many people fail to find material success, just because they are so convinced that they don't deserve it. Buttercup makes clear that superficial success or status is just part of the passing landscape, and that what matters is the relationship of the traveller to himself and to his journey.

Calendula Calendula officinalis

Positive: warmth.
Negative: lack of receptivity, sharpness.
Calendula, the pot marigold, is well known in herbal and homoeopathic medicine as a healer of cuts. The flower essence heals mental cuts – those inflicted by a sharp tongue. Too many people hide their 'heart of gold' behind an abrupt and scornful manner which causes great pain to others. They do themselves no favours, since that manner is based on fear that being nice to people makes one vulnerable to humiliating rejection. Calendula helps us dare to be kind.

California Poppy Escholzia Californica

Positive: discrimination.
Negative: distracted by 'fool's gold'.
The signature of *Escholzia* is its colour, the richest gold found in the flower kingdom. Light can either help us to see, or merely dazzle. *Escholzia* is a remedy for those who think they are seeing when they have been blinded by glitter. This can occur in the sense of a search for truth being sidetracked into involvement with drugs, cults and gurus – or of a whole life being distracted by the material glitter of 'high society'. Either way, the essence is said to restore balance to one's sense of values.

California Wild Rose Rosa Californica
Positive: caring, giving.
Negative: apathy.
The Bach Wild Rose is also characterised by apathy, but it is generally thought of as a state which is sad for the individual rather than affecting anyone else. In the California essence the essentially negative and destructive quality of apathy is made clear: apathy is the absence of love, and is therefore fundamentally anti-life. If you love and care you cannot be apathetic – the two things are opposites. 'In order for evil to triumph it is only necessary that good men do nothing', which begs the question, how can anyone who does nothing be called good? Wild Rose (both forms) is, therefore, all about taking responsibility for ourselves and the world we live in – if we can overcome apathy sufficiently to take it.

Camphor Cinnamomum camphora
Camphor, as used in mothballs etc. and in allopathic medicine, is generally regarded by homoeopaths as a menace, able to de-activate remedies in the bottle and antidote them in the patient. The flower essence is said to neutralise this effect (and that of coffee, the other homoeopathic *bête noire*) to some extent and to cleanse the system of other contaminations so as to make it more receptive to other remedies.

Chamomile Anthemis cotula
Positive: serenity.
Negative: dissatisfaction.
Chamomile in homoeopathic form is one of the essential childhood remedies, indicated for teething pains, colic and associated temper tantrums and whining. The flower essence addresses the same picture, possibly in a deeper,

subtler way. The chamomile child screams to have something and then throws it away when given: nothing pleases. In adult life, how often do we strive and yearn for some possession, some accomplishment, only to find that it does not satisfy, so that we end up like that small child, disappointed and frustrated? The chamomile essence can perhaps help us to grow up at last, to seek only what we value and to value what we have.

Chaparral Larrea Sp

Positive: balanced awareness.
Negative: inner disturbance.

The greatest problem of modern urban life is the degree of over-stimulation of the nervous system. Simply in terms of people, traffic, noise, there is too much to take in, which leads to all kinds of functional and dynamic disorders. Naturally, we go to great lengths to make matters worse, by watching sensational fantasies made into films and TV shows, and reading newspapers full of lurid accounts of bizarre events. With the result that we acquire the proverbial 'mind like a sewer'. Computer programmers used to say GINGO: Garbage In – Garbage Out. The human brain suffers rather more than a computer from an excess input of garbage since it does not have the facility to delete useless information. There is a lot to be said, then, for being rather careful about what we let through the door of our minds. Realistically, though, this is only likely to affect the rate at which the garbage piles up rather than standing a chance of stopping it, so a remedy which can at least partially cleanse our thoughts is worth knowing about. Chaparral may sound as though it would act on the same areas as a mixture of White Chestnut with Crab Apple. The big difference is that a lot of the White Chestnut chunter is generated from inside, whereas Chaparral is wholly

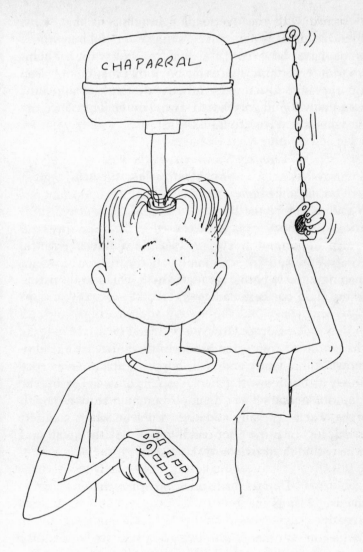

.... WATCHING SENSATIONAL FANTASIES
WE ACQUIRE THE PROVERBIAL 'MIND LIKE A SEWER'

concerned with the overloading impressions that come from outside. It is particularly suitable for children whose minds have been contaminated by excessive or inappropriate entertainments to the point that they do not sleep and appear to lose interest in what we think of as reality, but equally for adults who are aware of the junk cluttering their minds and wish to be rid of it.

Comfrey *Symphytum officinale*

Comfrey has been known from earliest times as a great herb for mending bones, so much so that it is important not to take it before the bone is held straight or it will heal crooked! In homoeopathy it is used in the same way, and is also important in eye injuries. As a flower essence, Comfrey is said to act mainly on the nervous system, opening up new pathways for growth where brain tissue, for example, has been damaged.

Cotton *Gossypium Arboreum*

The cotton of commerce produces the finest natural fibre known to humanity and, as it happens, makes an essence closely associated with hair. Questions of vanity apart, the condition of one's hair is an important pointer to the health of the system generally, and inner problems which manifest as hair loss or cause poor condition of the hair are all said to be within the province of this essence.

Dandelion *Taraxacum officinale*

Positive: relaxed energy.
Negative: tense, driven.
Dandelion, in other forms, is a good laxative so it is easy to see how in its more refined form it will work in a similar way on the mind. Its action is very similar to that of Vervain in the Bach series.

Deer Brush *Ceanothus integerrimus* (white)
Positive: clarity of purpose.
Negative: lack of awareness of unconscious motives.

Dill *Anethum Graveolens*
Positive: able to experience and use life's impressions to the full.
Negative: over-stimulation, hyper-sensitivity.
This is closely related in action to Chaparral (see above). Whereas Chaparral appears to act primarily to cleanse and avoid damage, Dill goes a step further in positively embracing a rich diversity of sensory experience and using it for positive development of the self.

Dogwood *Cornus nuttallii*
Positive: 'harmony with the body'.
Negative: awkwardness, physical self-consciousness.
Cornus Nuttallii is by far the most beautiful member of the highly attractive cornus family, so it is an appropriate essence to encourage ease and grace. Abuse in childhood engenders self-hatred, even to the point of self-mutilation, so that the victim never really feels at home in the body, with catastrophic results for the entire life. In a less extreme way this is an important essence for growing adolescents as they grow through the 'ugly duckling' phase and have to come to terms with all the physical and emotional changes involved in growing up.

Evening Primrose *Oenothera hookeri*
Positive: warmth, commitment.
Negative: repression, lack of commitment.
The ability to enter fully into a committed relationship with another human being is crucial to most people's happiness, yet many never manage it. Many a promising relationship

develops up to a point, but something stops it fulfilling its promise. The problem is usually cyclic and the script most often goes like this: 'Because I have been hurt/let down/ disappointed before, I won't commit myself until I'm really sure, just in case, then if it does go wrong I won't feel I've lost so much. If I see it going wrong, I can even get in first and be the one to walk away: that way at least I feel I'm in control.' Whether this takes the form of going in for multiple relationships (so as to provide a 'back-up' in case one doesn't work out) or simply going cold, to the bafflement and then fury of even the most patient partner, doesn't really matter. The result is always the same. The prophecy fulfils itself, another failure is added to the list and the cycle perpetuates and reinforces itself.

Anyone who is aware of being caught in this trap will need to do a great deal of conscious work on themselves and may need the help of a skilled therapist, but the essence may well help, crucially, to make the desired change in outlook.

Fairy Lantern Calochortus albus
Positive: acceptance of adult responsibilities.
Negative: eternal child.
Some people need encouraging to be child-like, in some respects: others need a lot of help to grow up. The greatest responsibility for any parent is to ensure that their progeny grow into adults. For a healthy individual this is no problem and indeed it is a great joy, but parents who have themselves been damaged or denied in some way are likely to mistake the purpose of having children altogether. In the same way that many people see marriage as an end rather than a beginning, very many parents think in terms of 'having a baby' in order to satisfy some need of theirs, rather than of bringing a soul into the world and taking

responsibility for helping it to incarnate to maturity. They become addicted to the power of having someone depend on them and resent rather than rejoice in any move of the dependent needy child towards independence.

If the child is strong as well as lucky, it will break away and 'only' suffer from guilt about this 'ungrateful' (in fact, perfectly natural) behaviour. If less lucky and less self-possessed, it will learn that love and approval are only obtained by remaining in a state of helpless dependency and simply refuse to grow up. Some stay all their lives with their parents and never marry, so that at least the mischief is not passed on. Many more do marry, but remain under the domination of the parent and unconsciously revenge themselves by inflicting the same pattern on their partner and children, so ensuring that the virus is passed on.

This essence is said to be appropriate not only for the condition described, but for all states of retardation in physical or emotional growth. It relates to a number of the Bach remedies – both Chicory and Centaury could apply in different phases, but this one is the specific for this very common and intractable problem. This suggests very forcefully the need for the use of flower essences to stop being an obscure specialism and to become integrated fully into the mainstream, in this case, of family therapy.

Golden Eardrops Dicentra chrysantha
Positive: in touch with and able to reconcile the past.
Negative: ailments from past events where the memory is suppressed.
Nobody likes pain and nobody likes remembering pain. Because it makes a deep impression, if we want to forget pain we must work pretty hard at it. Pain inflicted by those you love, and who are supposed to love you, hurts twice as

much so you have to work twice as hard to forget it. It is really important to forget it though, because the existence of the pain contradicts the love you are all supposed to feel and the contradiction is unbearable. And in fact, you can't really forget at all – as I mentioned before one of the improvements in the human condition had our brains been designed by IBM would have been the 'erase' button. But all you can do is bury the pain very deep inside and pretend you've forgotten it. Pretty much like the way we take all our toxic waste and dig a big hole in the ground to bury it in and then plant trees on top and call it a park and forget that it's really a rubbish dump. That is until the trees turn brown and the water goes a peculiar colour. So sooner or later, you have to dig it all up and see what's there, and do what you should have done to start with – dispose of it properly, safely and carefully. When that time comes in your emotional life the Golden Eardrops may be helpful.

Golden Rod *Solidago canadensis*
Positive: able to maintain individuality.
Negative: over-influenced by the group.

Golden Yarrow *Achillea clytedata*
Positive: ability to project the self, without coarsening.
Negative: losing self, or 'hardening' to protect.

These two important essences are quite closely related in nature as well as name and appearance. The Golden Yarrow is especially suited to people of an artistic or delicate sensibility who find it difficult to deal with the 'normal' world. Their reactions tend to polarise: either they withdraw into a Violet-like state so as to avoid the coarse contact, or else they put on a mask, a social persona, which is completely at odds with their inner nature. Although this works well enough in its way as a survival device, it causes

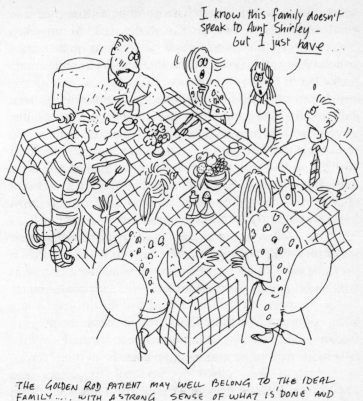

THE GOLDEN ROD PATIENT MAY WELL BELONG TO THE IDEAL FAMILY ..... WITH A STRONG SENSE OF WHAT IS 'DONE' AND 'NOT DONE'

difficulties with intimate relationships and also means that the world at large does not benefit from what should be a very definite influence for good. The Golden Yarrow strengthens and removes fear a person may have about letting other people see their true nature.

In the case of Golden Rod, the danger is less of masking the personality, more of losing it altogether. The Golden Rod patient may well belong to the ideal family, loving and strongly supportive of one another – and also subtly controlling of every action. There will be a strong sense of what is 'done' and 'not done', a whole series of unspoken (or even proudly proclaimed) injunctions and taboos which one cannot break in the smallest detail and remain a member of the loving supportive etc., etc.

It is not only families that operate in this way – social peer groups and even whole nations (not just communist ones either) operate in exactly the same way. It is also noticeable that the families and groups that operate most strongly in this way will be the most critical of any child who appears to 'follow the crowd' – if it is a different crowd. And it is those children who are precisely most likely to fall into sheep-like group behaviour: they will try to break away and assert their individuality, but because they are already crippled by their conditioning the furthest they can get is to join another group. (This, incidentally, is why street gang culture, with the most rigid and bizarre codes, becomes universal in a rigid and traditional society such as Japan.) The thing that distinguishes humans from the bees and badgers is the ability to be individual – to take part in the group but also to stand aside from it or even go against it at will, based on personal conscience and intelligence. If this is denied, we either turn into some form of fascist, or suffer great damage from the denial that this is a problem.

As with many essences, and with all therapy, the hardest thing with this one is to get the people who are in most need to realise their need to take it. The therapist is always painfully aware of nibbling around the edges of a situation because the only people who undertake treatment are those who are sufficiently aware of the problem to seek help, and who are therefore on the point of solving it anyway. However, if the essence helps to strengthen those who do try to break away, being confronted by the challenge this presents may have an indirect influence on the group as a whole.

Hibiscus *Hibiscus Sp*
Positive: integration of sexuality (female).
Negative: inability to connect sex with love.

Indian Paintbrush *Castilleja miniata*
Positive: energetic creativity.
Negative: devitalisation, exhaustion from creative effort.
This is closely related to Blackberry, in the ability or inability to see a project through. The Blackberry tendency is that the thing doesn't happen because it remains too much in the head. The Indian Paintbrush situation is a stage further on: the project is, as it were, given birth, but the effort involved leads to complete exhaustion. The condition is similar to the Bach Olive, but this essence is specified by the reason for the problem as well as its nature.

Iris *Iris douglasiana*
Iris deals with another aspect of creative exhaustion (very creative, these Californians!). This is not so much the exhaustion of the body as the drying up of inspiration, perhaps in other to save itself from the Indian Paintbrush state. The body closes down the flow of energy to the creative areas: unfortunately that energy is vital to its own well-being, too – we do not live by bread alone – so it will starve itself unless the situation is rebalanced.

Lavender *Lavandula officinalis*
Positive: refined awareness.
Negative: spiritual/mental over-stimulation – physical depletion.
The essential oil of Lavender is well known as a great aid

to relaxation and, as with so many other plant remedies, the flower essence shows the same characteristic raised to a higher plane. At the present time many people are rediscovering esoteric practices such as yoga and meditation and becoming very interested in working with spiritual energies. Some seem not to realise just how powerful these energies are, nor that it is far easier to open yourself up than to close off and protect yourself. In the old schools a student would have many years of training in 'self defence' before being allowed to attempt these practices but in the Western world, where the individual will is law, a number of people are having to find out for themselves that becoming open to energies that you have not learnt to control is actually very dangerous, both to physical health and mental stability.

There are also some people who are just naturally extremely sensitive to their surroundings and 'pick up' energy without intending to or even being aware of it. These people need to become conscious of what is happening and to learn to control it.

In both these cases, Lavender is said to help repair the worst of the damage and to assist in gaining the desired control.

Madia *Madia Elegans*

Positive: precision, focused attention.
Negative: dullness, inability to concentrate.
In order to learn we need to be open to all sorts of things. In order to produce, we need to be able to close off to some extent, to narrow the focus and stick to the task in hand. The person in need of Madia has difficulty in moving from the one mode to the other, and so finds it difficult to be productive. The essence is said to help control the focus so that one can 'open' and 'close' as appropriate.

Manzanita Arctostaphylos viscida

Positive: integration of spiritual and physical.
Negative: ascetic disgust at the body.

In the past a number of spiritual disciplines have made a point of 'mortifying the flesh'. Asceticism has been considered a virtue, even when monks and yogis would starve themselves to the point of emaciation. This is a mistaken point of view, since it can only shorten the physical life span and presumably the point of having a physical incarnation is to live through it as productively as possible. We have plenty of time to exist as pure spirit – in this physical world we act through the physical body, and this is made easier if we relate to that body with love. The Bach rubrics for Crab Apple touch this condition but cannot be said to address it fully. The Manzanita essence encourages a more balanced frame of mind in which the spirit is seen as being able to act in co-operation with the physical rather than being opposed to it.

Morning Glory Impomoea purpurea

Positive: awake, in touch.
Negative: not awake – out of touch.

Morning glory is indicated for people whose sleep patterns have become chronically disturbed with consequences for their general health. There is for each of us a proper and healthy balance of day and night-time activity. People who crave activity at night, whether it be 'clubbing' or computer hacking, quickly run out of natural energy and replace it by the use of various drugs. (There is a special brand of Cola marketed to insomniac computer enthusiasts which proudly proclaims that it contains three times as much caffeine as any other!) If this behaviour is sustained for long, it becomes impossible to settle back into a normal rhythm and one becomes sick and more and more detached from reality (I know, I've done it). Morning glory is said to make the rebalancing trick possible and restore the undead to life. With that name, what else could it do?

Mountain Pennyroyal *Monardella odoratissima** *
Positive: mental integrity and clarity.
Negative: influenced from outside.
Another of the remedies for those 'under the influence' – of what, in this case? Cerato as you may remember is influenced by other people's opinions. Golden Rod is under the collective thumb of the peer group. Lavender is detrimentally influenced by what we can only call raw energy. Now, Mountain Pennyroyal is for those influenced by the negative energies of those around them. Possibly by individual people, like Cerato, but not by what they say so much as the way they feel and the kind of energy they give off. Equally, it could be by the group, like Golden Rod, although again it is not so much the rules as the feelings and energy around them that will disturb. Or, somewhat like Lavender, it could be a disembodied energy, but not in this case abstract power but an individual entity which will attack and attempt to possess anyone who allows themself to become vulnerable, perhaps by unwise esoteric practices or the use of drugs.

In sum, this is said to help those who, for whatever reason, might feel that their mind is not altogether their own.

Mountain Pride *Penstemon newberryi*
Positive: moral courage.
Negative: not standing up for beliefs.
When Christ was arrested and taken for trial, his disciples were fearful of their lives and, as he foretold, denied all knowledge and connection with the man they had, only a

day before, enthusiastically hailed as their Lord and Saviour. Most of us, if put to far smaller tests, fail just as miserably. It is so easy to acquiesce in sexist, racist and generally obnoxious saloon bar banter and so hard to risk the ridicule of your companions by suggesting that they talk in a way fitting to adult humans. It is so tempting even to cover up what you do for a living lest a stranger should think you even a bit odd. How many of us then would stand up for a single victim against a baying crowd?

Not one – so we needn't be proud, but we do need to think how we could do even a little better. While writing this part of the book I read an account of the Australian journalists who stayed in East Timor to witness the Indonesian invasion and were butchered with insane cruelty by Indonesian soldiers just for being there. They felt that they owed it to the native victims of the invasion to witness and if possible report what happened, while the 'democratic' governments who armed the butchers resolutely looked the other way, as they still do. If we all had just a small fraction of that willingness to be sacrificed for right, would the world not be different? Think of the areas in your life where a little courage is called for and think whether this essence might help you.

Mullein *Verbascum Thapsis*
Positive: strong conscience.
Negative: confused, amoral.
Another 'moral' remedy, Mullein is concerned with the choices that govern our actions. Moral certainty is in short supply these days, as we make the transition from the childish state of accepting the rules laid down from above to accepting the adult responsibility for making our own decisions. This should not be thought of as an easy way out: we can do as we please, but only pleasing to do what

works will make us whole and happy. Many people systematically lie and cheat and deceive, making themselves thoroughly miserable in the process, but carrying on because they do not have the courage to change. It is only when conscience forces them to admit that their way of life is not working for them that a change will have to come. Nothing can make the decisions that we have to take easy, but if we can hear a clear voice of conscience, we can at least be more sure when we have chosen right.

Nasturtium Tropaeolum Majus

Positive: warmth, vitality.

Negative: depletion of energy from excessive intellectual activity.

Real health demands a balance of the elements that make up the individual – physical, mental, emotional and spiritual. If the intellect is over-developed or over-used at the expense of the other elements, great damage is done to the individual and to society. This essence is appropriate on a short-term basis for anyone who finds themselves feeling 'not right' after a bout of mental exertion – revising for exams, or writing a book, perhaps. It is also suitable for the more chronic state of children whose intellectual development has been hot-housed: the indications of retarded emotional and physical development will be very clear. Nasturtium can be compared but not confused with Indian Paintbrush. The Indian Paintbrush exhaustion is from creativity, pouring oneself into the painting, symphony, whatever. Nasturtium gets it more from a hard, not particularly rewarding slog over the law reports or the accounts. The need for this essence is likely to increase at the present time with the return to competitiveness and the application of purely intellectual standards in popular education.

Oregon Grape Berberis aquifolium
Positive: positive expectations of others.
Negative: paranoia, negative projection.
Healthy children instinctively assume that everyone in the world is, at least potentially, a friend and ally. By adulthood, many people have formed the conclusion that, with a few exceptions, the world is hostile and full of enemies. How does this happen? It is true that the child has to learn not to trust everyone implicitly – unfortunately, this lesson tends to be taught by scare campaigns which give the impression that any unknown adult is a threat (which ignores the fact that, for all the publicity given to sensational abductions and murders, most violence against children is perpetrated within the family).

Adults who regard an approaching newcomer with a relaxed smile still exist, though they are becoming rare, while there are many whose automatic reaction to any new situation is the threat of violence. Anger breeds hate and love breeds kindness so the vicious spiral has to be broken and reversed. Once again, the essence will not be taken by those who most need it, but if those who are aware recognise the traces of this behaviour and work on it in themselves, the virus of kindness will spread, slowly but inevitably.

Penstemon Penstemon davidsonii
Positive: bears difficulties with fortitude.
Negative: self-pity.
All lives have periods of sadness and difficulty: these are the challenges and lessons which shape our development and give us the opportunity to become adult humans instead of spoilt children. Some people are less willing to see things this way and, rather than learning their lessons, complain at the unfairness of it all. Transforming that point of view

cannot be done without personal work, but this essence may help those who are striving to see positive purpose in the hardships of life. There is a relationship with the Bach Willow: I would distinguish them by saying that Willow's complaining is often from relatively trivial causes. Penstemon is really for those undergoing the major challenges which make it easy to justify the negative state, but all the more important that it be overcome.

Peppermint Mentha piperita

Positive: Clarity.

Negative: Mental sluggishness.

This is a complementary essence to Nasturtium. In Nasturtium excessive mental activity weakens the body. In the Peppermint patient, excessive energy demands from the vegetative parts – digestion and liver – deplete the mental energy, making it difficult to think clearly, especially after a meal. They will find that their mind works best when they are a little hungry, but that mental activity stimulates the hunger until they are overtaken by the urge to eat something, at which point the mental energy collapses. Since they are often engaged in demanding and important work it will be evident that this kind of imbalance makes enormous dents in creative output, so that it is not only unpleasant but also expensive and well worth correcting.

Pink Monkeyflower Mimulus lewisii

Positive: emotional honesty.

Negative: hides feelings from sense of shame.

This important 'heart' remedy is a member of the *Mimulus* family. The Bach Mimulus is general for any identifiable fear. This deals specifically with the fears of those who have experienced rejection and humiliation and are afraid to 'expose' themselves in any sense. They may be actually shy

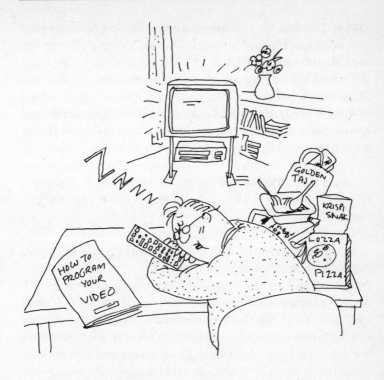

IN THE PEPPERMINT PATIENT MENTAL ACTIVITY
STIMULATES HUNGER UNTIL THEY ARE
OVERTAKEN BY AN URGE TO EAT SOMETHING
AT WHICH POINT THE MENTAL ENERGY
COLLAPSES

and reclusive, avoiding any kind of contact with others, or
they may behave in a cold and guarded way, dressing,
wearing their hair, using spectacles in a way that 'covers
them from view'. It is well indicated for survivors of abuse,
but abuse takes many forms, not only physical molestation.
Many children who have never been physically interfered
with nonetheless grow up with a deep sense of shame and
inadequacy in relation to their sexuality and emotions,

instilled by mockery or insinuation – nothing concrete that can be uncovered or 'proved', but no less real. Being left with this sense that there is no basis for feeling the way you do unless you really are dirty, unworthy, etc., makes the condition terribly difficult to deal with, which is why I personally regard this as the most insidious and pernicious form of abuse, although it is one for which no one will ever be prosecuted. However we work to process the past, the urgent need is to be able to overcome the feeling in the present, to allow ourselves to make contact and form relationships which will heal, and that is the purpose of this essence.

Pink Yarrow *Achillea millefolium* var, *rubra*

Positive: clear emotional boundaries.
Negative: lack of boundaries, takes on others' 'junk'.
To be sensitive to the needs and cares of others is a great and necessary gift. To be oversensitive to the extent that one becomes a 'sponge', soaking up whatever is around, to the confusion and detriment of an emotional life of one's own, is not so good. This essence will apply to a number of adults who might otherwise be treated with remedies such as Centaury or Red Chestnut. But it will be especially important for children, where tension and emotional difficulty exist among the adults in the household, since, even if not consciously aware of the problem, a child will absorb the emotional 'vibration' and reflect it in some aspect of his or her own behaviour, or even by becoming seriously ill.

Pomegranate *Punica granatum*

Positive: (female) integration of aspects of life.
Negative: (female) confusion about role.
This is very much a remedy for the modern woman.

Innumerable books and magazine articles are written giving conflicting advice about how best to reconcile the demands of career, lover/husband, home-making and children: all wasted, because there is no 'right' answer. Women clearly have more choices available to them and have to take the responsibility for designing a life plan, rather than accepting one out of the box. Since this always involves compromise, there is always likely to be room for feelings of guilt about whichever aspect has been given a low priority, and the exploitation of that guilt is both profitable and popular.

Perhaps what is really needed is to get clear that one does not have to behave in this or that way in order to be a 'real' woman: every woman is as real as any other, regardless of how she chooses to live her life. If the essence helps achieve that sort of perspective so that whatever decisions are taken as an individual do not appear to threaten or undermine the feminine identity, it will save a great deal of unhappiness and confusion.

Rabbitbrush Chrysothamnus nauseosus

Positive: mental flexibility: integration of central and peripheral.
Negative: polarisation of mental processes.
This is a remedy dear to my heart since my work as a vision educator is largely based on the need to see central focus and peripheral awareness as two aspects of the same thing and not as two different things. It is important, not only for vision, but for all learning: in reading, for instance, one must take in each letter and word, while integrating them into the overall context. In playing football, one must give absolute attention to the location of the ball while remaining aware of the locations of other players and the possibilities of space between them. A surprising number of people, however,

turn out to lack the ability to integrate information in this way. The difficulty can be covered up when demands are small by switching back and forth between 'modes', but the problem shows up when a more taxing demand is made which is simply found impossible. It would not be an exaggeration to say that every case of every kind of learning difficulty that has come my way has involved this failing.

There are a number of well-established ways of working on this difficulty, ranging from the classical Bates vision work to state of the art kinesiology techniques. Use of the Rabbitbrush essence should enhance the effect of any work of this sort, and, in case of slight difficulty, may be sufficient by itself.

Saint John's Wort *Hypericum perforatum* *
Positive: illuminated consciousness.
Negative: 'over-expanded' consciousness.
Hypericum is an important member of the homoeopathic armoury, where it is an important remedy for inflammation and nerve damage. Both of these areas can be related to the capacity to circulate energy through the body and the flower essence represents this idea in a more refined way, relating to the circulation of light throughout the organism. It is held to be an important protection remedy for those who are vulnerable to psychic attack and depletion (see also Lavender).

Scarlet Monkeyflower *Mimulus Cardinalis*
Positive: emotional honesty.
Negative: fear of intense feelings, of the 'dark side'.
This is closely related to the Pink Monkeyflower, showing another aspect of emotional fear. People who have been taught that the expression of anger is not acceptable learn to 'stuff' their feelings until they either slowly poison

themselves or the lid blows off with the suddenness and force of a human Krakatoa. Any such explosion is, of course, extremely frightening and leads to a redoubling of the effort to put the lid back on.

It also happens that *any* strong emotion, positive as well as negative, is viewed with the same suspicion, which leads to a generally repressed state and complete inability to communicate on a feeling level. It is vital for such people to learn to acknowledge and examine these deep and power-ful feelings, and to let them out when necessary: this may also involve re-educating those around into slightly differ-ent expectations.

Sticky Monkeyflower Mimulus aurantiacus

Positive: integration of warmth and intimacy.
Negative: sexuality disconnected from feeling.
This is one of a number of essences connected with the integration of sexuality with feeling. Hibiscus deals broadly with the same area, but is specifically suitable for women; Basil deals with the connection between sex and the spiritual aspect of love; whereas this essence is focused on the connection between sex and ordinary warmth and affection. I once heard it said, half jokingly, that women give sex in order to obtain affection and men give affection in order to obtain sex. If there is truth in this it is extremely sad since the giving and receiving of both aspects at once is the most rewarding experience most of us are likely to have. If this is an area that needs work, it might be a good idea to begin with this essence for a period, and to work on building a firm basis of physical and emotional warmth and trust, before using Basil to help explore the 'higher' regions.

Sweet Pea Lathyrus latifolius

Positive: finding one's place.

Negative: social alienation.

At one time the nomadic way of life was confined to those whose environments would not support a long stay in one place. With the development of settled communities it became commonplace for whole generations to be born, grow up and die within a mile of the same spot. In the present age, for various reasons, it is rapidly becoming unusual for children to settle in the same county as their parents, let alone the same street, and just as unusual for anyone to live a whole life span in one place. As with other aspects of life, it is now open to most of us to make a choice as to where we want to be rather than allowing the choice to be made for us, and together with the advantages of this there are considerable problems. Both for the nomadic hippy traveller and the executive who buys a house from a brochure in a scenic commuter village, there are the twin difficulties of having no established basis for social relations and no feeling of belonging to a place.

This has to be resolved, either by accepting our lot as pilgrims, and carrying our 'home' inside us as we roam from place to place, or by finding the right place to 'put down our roots' and staying there. Whichever is the appropriate choice, this essence is said to help in making it and in establishing the sense of home, wherever it may be.

Trumpet Vine *Campsis tagliabuana*
Positive: verbal expressiveness.
Negative: inarticulate, speech difficulties.

This gorgeous climbing plant has flaming orange/red flowers (indicating its outgoing qualities) in a shape rather reminiscent of a megaphone or gramophone horn.

In my earlier career as a music teacher, I discovered at first hand the intimate connection between the use of the

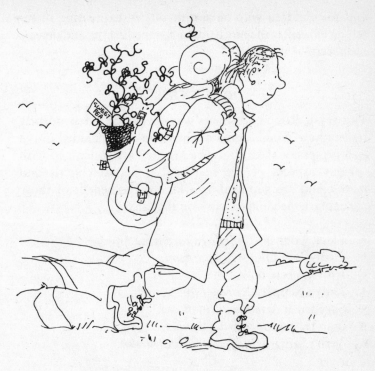

SWEET PEA ..... HELPS IN ESTABLISHING
A SENSE OF HOME, WHEREVER IT MAY BE..

voice and the feeling of self. Conditions that at first sight appeared to be of entirely physical origin turned out to have recognisable and predictable connections to the inner emotional life. There is a close connection then between this essence and the Pink Monkeyflower since one of the most common ways we attempt to hide or disguise our-selves is through the way we project, or fail to project, ourselves through the voice. This essence could be thought of as appropriate, among others, for those who find difficulty in speaking in public, with a dull, dry delivery, and for children who have difficulty in expressing themselves, as well as the more obvious impediments and defects of speech.

THE SEVEN HERBS

This small group of essences was developed independently by Mathew Wood. Some of them are also included in the FES professional kit, but as a set they are concerned with various aspects of the relationship between spirit and matter and are supplied as a kit for the benefit of those particularly needing to work on that area.

- Black Cohosh *Cimicifuga racemosa*.
- Easter Lily *Lilium longiflorum*.
- Iris *Iris versicolor*.
- Lady's Slipper *Cypripedium parviflora*.
- Sagebrush *Artemisia tridentata*.
- Star Tulip *Calochortus tolmiei*.
- Yerba Santa *Eriodyction californicum*.

7

The Australian Bush essences

ORIGINS

The Australian Bush flower essences in their contemporary, commercial form were created in the 1980s by Ian White. Ian represents the fifth generation of a family tradition of herbal medicine, although he originally planned to follow a different path. He studied psychology at university but found that the teachings of natural health practitioners seemed to carry more enlightenment about the workings of the human mind than the academic theories he learned in school, so he studied and trained as a naturopath after all and became a highly respected practitioner and teacher in his own right.

The severe illness of a dear friend prompted him to participate in a healing meditation circle and it was during these meditations that he began to 'see' visions of flowers, together with information about how they could be used in healing. By a curious synchronicity, very often immediately after the 'channelling' of a new remedy in this way, he was presented with a patient suffering from an appropriate problem for testing it out. He found that in every case the therapeutic result confirmed the 'channelled' description and in this way he began to collect remedies and bring them into use. He subsequently took great trouble to cross-check the descriptions by scientific and esoteric means and found absolute confirmation from every source.

Ian's book, *Australian Bush Flower Essences*, is indispensable reading not only for anyone wanting to know these remedies but for anyone with any kind of interest in plants or healing. It describes 50 remedies in great detail together with beautiful line drawings and excellent coloured photographs of the plants.

Australia is one of the world's larger and more remote islands, with a marvellous diversity of plant and animal life which has evolved in unique forms as a result of its isolation. Despite mass extinctions since the coming of 'civilisation', the Australian bush contains thousands if not millions of life forms unknown anywhere else. It also contains one of the most ancient surviving human cultures. The Australian aboriginals were despised as savages by the early white settlers, and have not fared particularly well since, yet theirs is in many ways a learned and refined culture far superior to our own. Merely to survive in the rigorous environment of the bush, without shelter, plumbing or clothing is far beyond the inner resources of most white people, yet the aborigines have been making themselves extremely comfortable there for thousands of years. Part of their learning is an extensive lore of plants and their uses, which included the value of healing essences made from flowers although, according to Ian White, that knowledge was much greater a few centuries ago.

CHARACTER

Australia, like America, is a country which is at once both young and ancient. The aboriginal culture combines profound practicality with deep spirituality, both coming from the extreme closeness to the earth. The new population, for similar reasons, could be said to combine practical self-confidence, to the point of brashness, with a growing longing to confront deeper questions.

These characteristics are strongly reflected in the general flavour of the Bush essences, which address the physical and the meta-physical in one breath. It has been pointed out that the high proportion of red and purple flowers in the Australasian flora, together with the range of exotic and bizarre forms, suggests a strong focus on sexuality and this is certainly the case. The Australian essences address the issues of healing relationships and sexuality in all its dimensions very directly and candidly.

Anyone at all put off by the complex and varied reference points of the California remedies will feel much more at home with the Bush essences. Like the Bach remedies, the descriptions are almost entirely based on emotional characteristics. They do, however, resemble the California remedies in drawing more specific pictures, relating emotions to particular situations. Many of the remedies present a complex picture, referring to several elements which are looked for in combination. To the experienced Bach user this might seem to restrict their application: on the other hand, it means that where there is a good fit to the situation, a single Bush essence may serve in a case which would require a collection of Bach remedies – you have a choice.

PRESCRIBING AND WORKING WITH
THE ESSENCES

Ian White prefers to cross-check prescriptions by muscle testing. For anyone who has the skills of kinesiology this is obviously worth while in order to check priority ('This is the most important area to correct now') and acceptability ('This body will accept this remedy now') and so on. However, the emotional pictures are sufficiently clearly drawn to make it possible to prescribe confidently from interview keynotes, just as with the Bach remedies, and the lack of muscle testing skill should not put anyone off using these remedies.

The dosage regime is rather different from the standard Bach method. The dose is 'seven drops on rising and retiring for two weeks'. This should be followed closely for best results. It is strongly suggested that working with affirmations which support the action of the essences will be most helpful.

THE DESCRIPTIONS

As with the California essences I have confined full descriptions to those where I have something to say! This is, however, a full listing of the Bush essences, at least by name and keynote. Where I have drawn comparisons with remedies of the other groups, this should not be thought of as being dismissive, implying that one is better or worse, or that it would make no difference which is used. On the contrary, if working with one of the particular problems which offers a choice of remedies, I would suggest very close and careful differential diagnosis to select the one that will work best in the individual case. Careful comparison and contrasting of the original descriptions of closely related remedies is actually the best way to really appreciate the uniqueness of each.

Swamp Banksia *Banksia robur*

Positive: energy, enjoyment.
Negative: temporary loss of enthusiasm and energy, frustration, 'burnout'.
Among the Bach remedies the closest equivalents to this essence would be Elm (loss of enthusiasm) and Oak (failing strength). It also covers elements of Olive (exhaustion) and Impatiens (frustration). It also probably relates quite closely to people who, in the normal way, might be candidates for Vervain. A valuable single remedy for a common situation.

Bauhinia *Lisiphyllum cunninghamii*

Positive: acceptance of new ideas: open mind.
Negative: resistance to change, rigidity.
A good remedy, possibly, for those who have trouble accepting new remedies! To cover this definition with Bach remedies, one would have to look to Walnut for the general acceptance of change, possibly Honeysuckle for undue attachment to the past, and Beech, or maybe Vine, according to the individual for the element of criticism. With the rate of change of circumstances and ideas in the present age, maintaining the balance – neither being stuck in the old nor swept away with the new – is a trick worth acquiring. This suggests itself as an important remedy for the times.

Billygoat Plum *Planchonia careeya*

Positive: sexual pleasure, self-acceptance.
Negative: self-disgust, sexual revulsion.
This is clearly very close to the Bach Crab Apple. It is

entirely appropriate for general conditions of 'uncleanness' – especially skin complaints – but it also has a strong specific emphasis on sexual disgust. As well as people who have difficulty coming to terms with sexual feelings and acts in general, it is particularly indicated for survivors of rape and sexual abuse, who need to cleanse and reclaim their sexuality. The note of self-acceptance is crucial. No complaint, whether physical or mental can be healed while we are in a state of self-loathing.

Black-eyed Susan Tetratheca ericifolia
Positive: slowing down, inner peace.
Negative: stress, rushing.
Note that this is *not* the same plant as the California essence of the same name. The action of this essence covers that of both Impatiens and Vervain. Ian White says, 'This is *the* remedy for stress.'

Bluebell Wahlenbergia species
Positive: joyful, trusting.
Negative: emotionally closed, fears lack.
Fill a glass with water, drink half the water. Now look at it. Is the glass half empty or is it half full? Some people are driven by the fear that if they share or give anything away they will be left short. You see a certain kind of child at a birthday party anxiously piling his plate with food he has no intention of eating, just in case someone else gets more. You see people who discourage their partners from having other friends or interests in case they get left out. The Bluebell essence, like a few of the Australian set, is akin to the Bach remedies in that the *reason* for the feeling is not so particularly important as its quality. Whatever the reason, or the issue, if that inexplicable meanness comes into the picture, Bluebell will be indicated.

Boronia *Boronia ledifolia*
Positive: calm, clarity.
Negative: broken heart, obsession.
Boronia, on the other hand, is very much an issue remedy.
It has a general action which is very close to White
Chestnuts in clearing the mind from obsessive thoughts
and focusing on the present, but it is also quite specific to
the situation of a broken relationship – the 'can't get him/
her out of my mind' sort of thing.

Bottlebrush *Callistemon linearis*
Positive: ability to move on.
Negative: difficulty in adapting to life changes.
The effect of this essence would appear to be very close to
Walnut.

Bush Fuchsia *Epacris longifloria*
Positive: articulation, balance.
Negative: reading, learning and speech difficulties.
This essence appears very close in scope to the Californian
Trumpet Vine.

Bush Gardenia *Gardenia megasperma*
Positive: relationships rejuvenated.
Negative: stale relationships.
This essence is for those who have begun to take each other
for granted, or are otherwise getting out of touch with each
other. If not addressed, it can mean a marriage breaking up
for no good reason, or children and parents being need-
lessly estranged. One of the more distasteful sides to the
so-called 'New Age thinking' is the attitude that, because it
is accepted that relationships are not necessarily forever, it
is OK to move on as soon as there is the slightest friction
or loss of interest. Such ideas as commitment or making an

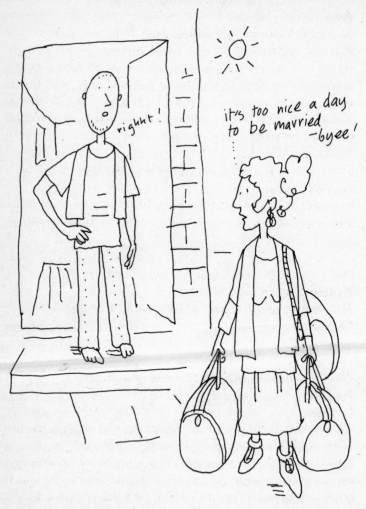

BUSH GARDENIA —
MARRIAGE BREAKING UP FOR NO
GOOD REASON . . . .

effort have been laughed at as ridiculously quaint and outmoded. A balanced view would suggest that, although of course there is no point in remaining in relationships that are unproductive, the old-fashioned virtues of constancy and fidelity have a lot going for them. No essence is going to make a dead relationship work, indeed, if things really are beyond repair I would expect using the essence would clarify feelings about the situation and help to find the way forward. But there are many relationships with plenty of life in them that are broken, just because they go a little off the rails and no one knows how to put them back on. Above all, the Bush Gardenia essence works by lifting us out of selfish self-absorption and helping us to actually see the other person, which is the essence of relationship.

Bush Iris *Patersonia longifolia*

Positive: assists transition.
Negative: fear of death.
The action of this essence appears very close to the Californian Angel's Trumpet.

Crowea *Crowea saligna*

Positive: centering.
Negative: worry.
Crowea is a great remedy for worry: it does not matter what about. This gives it a slightly tighter focus than, say White Chestnut, where the fullness of mind can be caused by a number of other things, but allows it to be prescribed confidently without needing exhaustive details. In fact a good indication is that the patient may well find it difficult to pinpoint the source of the worry. Often that is because there isn't one: a lot of worrying is just a habit, a rather scratchy gramophone record that we like to play to keep us company. If something worries you, ask: 'Can I do

anything about this problem?' If yes – do it at once, then there is no need to worry any more. If no – stop worrying and save your energy for dealing with real problems when they come. Easier said than done, but this essence will help.

Dagger Hakea Hakea teretifolia

Positive: forgiveness.
Negative: resentment, bitterness.

If to forgive is divine, the use of this essence can make us a little more like gods. It is easy to feel good about people who have been nice to you. But when someone has, perhaps, hurt you very badly, you not only do not feel good about them, you actively resist feeling good about them. You lock that hurt away and then get it out and gloat over it like an old war medal. Like most negative behaviour, this has little effect on the other party but it does a great deal of damage to you. The habit of nursing these wounds can only be overcome by determined personal work but the use of the essence will make it easier to accept the need to release and to carry it through.

Dog Rose Bauera rubioides

Positive: confidence.
Negative: shyness, fear.

Mimulus is fearful, of something; Aspen has nameless fears; Red Chestnut is fearful on behalf of others. Dog Rose is characterised by a generally fearful outlook on life – the Dog Rose patient seems almost to be looking for things to be afraid of. This has two effects: firstly it makes the feared things more likely to happen, and secondly it wastes a tremendous amount of energy. It also restricts one's activities, because the uppermost thought is always 'What if it goes wrong?' (cf the homoeopathic Argentum Nitricum).

This essence acts to rebalance the energies so that new activities can be undertaken with confidence, and life can be enjoyed as it should be.

Five Corners *Styphelia triflora*
Positive: self love.
Negative: low self-esteem.
This acts in a very similar way to the Californian Buttercup.

Flannel Flower *Actinotus helianthi*
Positive: openness, enjoyment of physical activity.
Negative: lack of sensitivity, dislike of touch.
This is an important remedy for men who have been brought up to equate any kind of sensuality with femininity, with the result that they use their bodies stiffly and avoid more than the most cursory contact with others – male or female. Their sex lives tend to be rather limited, since they do not enjoy real physical tenderness and always need to be in control to an excessive degree. There may be an association with physical abuse in childhood, or it may just be the cultural ideal of 'manhood' that causes the problem: either way it is important to learn that sensual enjoyment does not compromise one's masculinity. Although predominantly a 'male' remedy, it also works effectively for women where well indicated.

Fringed Violet *Thysanotus tuberosus*
Positive: reintegration.
Negative: effects of shock, trauma.
This essence covers broadly the same ground as Arnica (Cal. Hom.) and Star of Bethlehem (Bach).

Grey Spider Flower Grevillea buxifolia
Positive: calmness, faith.
Negative: terror.
This essence acts in a similar way to Rock Rose (Bach).

Hibbertia Hibbertia pendunculata
Positive: content, knowledge utilised.
Negative: fanatical self-improvement, knowledge acquired but not assimilated.

There are people, in this present age, for whom 'self-improvement' has become an end in itself, a self-sustaining craze. These people seem to vie with each other – who can do the most courses, read the most improving books, learn the most techniques. And yet, for all the money they invest and the hours they spend, they do not seem to be happier or healthier than anyone else. I remember taking a friend to a particular seminar (I used to do a bit of this myself) which I thought she would find interesting. As I was enjoying it, I asked her in a break how she found it and received a detailed lecture about how it was the same as this and not as good as that, as one might criticise a film. She got no benefit from the weekend at all, because she was so busy *knowing all about it* that she refused to be part of it. Unfortunately, I have seen the same thing at courses I have run, where some members are so busy being knowledge-able and knowing about the proceedings that they learn nothing.

This essence can also be used for people who are fanatical and inflexible in other ways: the indefatigably 'politically correct' come to mind for some reason. Ian White notes that the mental stiffness is often reflected in the body. I would add that this seems to affect the eyes particularly which would account for so many people of this cast of mind being long sighted.

The crucial issue is the difference between knowing all about something and knowing something in a way which is of practical use. The Bach remedies to compare are Vine, Cerato, Chestnut Bud.

Illawarra Flame Tree *Brachychiton acerifolius*
Positive: confidence.
Negative: fear of responsibility.
This essence is related in its action to Larch and Hornbeam (Bach). Such people hold back from developing their potential or from taking on any commitment in the hope of there being a 'better time' later. The essence helps them break out of this delusion and realise that the time to act is now.

Isopogon *Isopogon anethifolius*
Positive: learn from the past/flexible in relating.
Negative: poor memory/dominating.
There are two distinct aspects to this essence. It resembles Chestnut Bud (Bach) in the inability to learn from the past, and Vine (Bach) in its bossy and domineering attitude to others. The connection is, of course, that the poor memory makes it easy to conveniently forget the mistakes we have made and to hold on to the myth of our infallibility. If we remember accurately what actually happened, we tend to be a little more humble.

Jacaranda *Jacaranda mimosaefolia*
Positive: centred.
Negative: scattered.
The negative Jacaranda type is 'all over the place' rather like AA Milne's Tigger: bouncing around full of energy and always starting new projects which are quickly forgotten as the next thing comes along. In the positive phase they are

much more centred and able to follow through. There is still the same quickness of intelligence but it is stimulating rather than wearying, being directed to a clear purpose. Many Gemini people will need this essence.

Kangaroo Paw *Anigozanthos manglesii*

Positive: poised.
Negative: gauche, unaware.
Kangaroo Paw essence is for people lacking social graces: although full of good intentions they come across as clumsy and insensitive to others and are extremely uncomfortable as well as a source of embarrassment in social situations. It can also be applied to people who are prone to becoming flustered and self-conscious and also to those who are insensitive to others in different ways.

Kapok Bush *Cochlospermum fraseri*

Positive: application.
Negative: apathetic.
This essence has a broadly similar character to the Wild Roses (California and Bach).

Little Flannel Flower *Actinotus minor*

Positive: playfulness.
Negative: over-seriousness.
This is a remedy for those who need to rediscover the 'child within'. It applies both to adults who are so overtaken by the seriousness of life that they forget how to laugh and play, and to children who are 'old before their time'. It is not to the credit of our culture that having fun is supposed to be incompatible with doing anything useful: although sometimes the expectations are upended in a very public way. When Richard Branson, who, it is safe to say, is one of the more laid-back millionaires of our times, took British

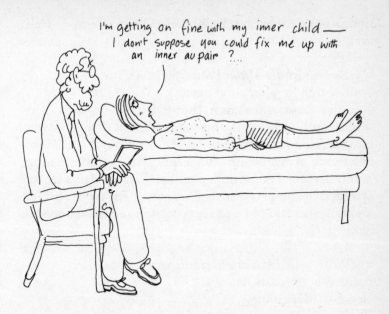

I'm getting on fine with my inner child —
I don't suppose you could fix me up with
an inner au pair?...

Airways to court, the 'serious' businessmen were taken
completely off guard. The chairman of BA later admitted
that he had obviously underestimated the opposition, but
that he could not have been expected to take the fellow
seriously because he was not wearing a grey suit. Some
Little Flannel Flower in the boardroom carafes at BA
would obviously be a help.

Macrocarpa *Eucalyptus macrocarpa*

Positive: vitality.
Negative: burnout.
Compare with Aloe Vera (California).

Mountain Devil *Lambertia formosa*

Positive: love.
Negative: hatred.

Compare with Holly (Bach) and Oregon Grape (California).

Mulla Mulla *Ptilotus atripicifolius*

Positive: regeneration after burns.
Negative: trauma from heat, fear of flames.
Mulla Mulla grows in the hottest part of the desert and can be thought of as symbolising the miraculous ability of vegetation to regenerate after a fire. The essence is said to be effective for healing both physical burns, whether recent or old, and the psychological effects of having been in a fire. It is also said to be effective against radiation and sun burning.

Old Man Banksia *Banksia serrata*

Positive: enthusiasm, energy.
Negative: sluggishness.
Compare with Peppermint (California).

Paw Paw *Carica papaya*

Positive: clarity, assimilation.
Negative: feeling overwhelmed.
The sense of being overwhelmed can have many causes. It can be the responsibility of making an important decision or taking on a big job, in which case one might consider Bach Elm; or it could be a mass of information that has to be taken in, or even a sudden and joyful event in life. If the thought that comes up is 'I can't handle it', consider Paw Paw.

Peach Flowered Tea Tree *Leptospermum squarrosum*

Positive: emotional stability, trust in health.
Negative: mood swings, hypochondria.
Peach Flowered Tea Tree is good for those who are

excessively preoccupied with their health and who are subject to swings of mood. They often lack consistency in following through projects, but in a different way from Jacaranda. Whereas Jacaranda, magpie-like, has his attention caught by the next thing that comes along, without any break in the relentless state of high energy, the Peach Flowered Tea Tree patient will start something with enthusiasm and then get bored and give it up because it no longer seems worth while – and may even sink into a Gentian-like (Bach) despondency. Although they are generally very capable people, this behaviour causes a lot of wasted effort and frustration, to themselves and those around them. With the aid of the essence they can become more balanced, productive and generally a great deal happier.

Philotheca Philotheca salsolifolia
Positive: ability to accept love and praise.
Negative: inability to accept praise or acknowledgement.
At bottom, everybody wishes to be loved and praised for their achievements. There is a balance to be struck: it is obviously undesirable to be so insecure that we cannot function without constant praise, but neither can we operate in a vacuum, without obtaining any kind of feedback from those around us. We are taught that it is wrong to 'blow our own trumpet' but there is no reason why we should feel the need to rush from the room with burning ears if someone else blows it for us. If we have worked and achieved, then a brief period of basking in the warmth of others' praise is part of our natural reward. If we are unable to accept that, we deprive ourselves of an important source of the energy that we need to go on, and also compromise our ability to praise and encourage others in turn. Although some would attempt to include this character under more general rubrics such as those for

Rock Rose or Water Violet, I feel that this needs to be recognised as a very distinct problem and that Ian White has done a great service by discovering this essence and elucidating its character.

Red Grevillea *Grevillea speciosa*
Positive: moving on.
Negative: stuck.
This essence is for people who feel stuck in their lives, and perhaps dominated by or dependent on someone else. The essence helps them to see that they are actually free to move and gives them the courage to act on this knowledge. The character relates in some ways to Cerato (Bach), but has this specific sense of moving on and out of the situation, whereas Cerato would focus more on changing the quality of relationships.

Red Helmet Orchid *Corybas dilatatus*
Positive: respectful, considerate.
Negative: rebellious, selfish.

Red Lily *Nelumbo nucifera*
Positive: grounded, focused.
Negative: spaced out, absent-minded.
This should not be confused with the condition of Fringed Violet (Australian Bush) or Arnica (California), both of which are definitely 'spaced out' but from a specific traumatic cause. This is far more akin to Clematis (Bach) or the homoeopathic Cannabis Indica. The person needing this essence will permanently give the sense of being 'not all there' – not in the sense of being unintelligent but of being unable to connect in any meaningful way to what is going on around them or to other people. It is often connected to a history of drug abuse, but can equally apply to a very

abstracted academic type – the archetypal 'mad professor' – and simply to anyone who has difficulty in getting their mind into focus on the task in hand – cf Hornbeam (Bach).

She Oak Casuarina glauca
Positive: (female) balance, fertility.
Negative: (female) hormonal imbalance, infertility.

Silver Princess Eucalyptus caesia
Positive: motivation.
Negative: aimlessness.
Silver Princess is for people who lack a sense of direction in their lives. At first sight, this essence might appear to duplicate the effect of Wild Oat (Bach), with perhaps a tinge of Gorse or Gentian for the feeling of hopelessness. But it is actually quite distinct since it deals, not only with finding the direction, but maintaining the sense of satisfaction and achievement when it is found and pursued. And what could be more important than finding and achieving our purpose?

Slender Rice Flower Pimelea linifolia
Positive: humility, open mind.
Negative: pride, narrow-mindedness.
This is a great essence for facilitating co-operation in every sphere. It helps people to see other sides of a question instead of rigidly defending their own corner. Used sufficiently widely it could bring politics to an end.

Southern Cross Xanthosia rotundifolia
Positive: responsibility.
Negative: resentment.
This essence bears comparison with Bluebell (Australian Bush) in that it covers poverty consciousness. However, the

character is, as ever, quite distinct. Whereas Bluebell is not actually deprived, but fears that he may be, Southern Cross suffers some deprivation, real or imagined, but instead of either doing something about it or appreciating what he has, blames the world and resents bitterly those who have or do more. This is quite close to the victim mentality of Willow (Bach), but is perhaps more specifically focused on the material aspects of life, whereas Willow's resentment could be as well triggered by a minor illness or the weather.

Spinifex Triodia species
Positive: healing through emotional understanding.
Negative: skin affections, herpes.
This is a powerful healer for skin affections, including fine cuts, but it is mainly concerned with the connection between the inner emotional state and what comes out on the surface.

Sturt Desert Pea Clianthus formosus
Positive: letting go.
Negative: pain, sadness.
This essence is for those who are trapped in the past by some deep hurt, especially from old love affairs. In this respect it is more specific than, say Honeysuckle (Bach) which is for the general attachment to the past. Whereas Dagger Hakea (Australian Bush) expresses anger and resentment about the hurt, Sturt Desert Pea has feelings of sadness and regret: in many situations the feelings will alternate so that the two essences could be used concurrently or successively as appropriate. Such a deep pain can keep one permanently off balance and cause long-standing physical ailments: it is yet another way that we become 'stuck' and block the natural flow of energy, so no

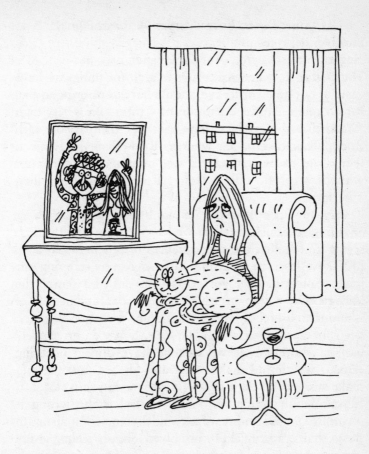

STURT DESERT PEA — THIS ESSENCE IS FOR
THOSE WHO ARE TRAPPED IN THE PAST BY
SOME DEEP HURT, ESPECIALLY FROM OLD
LOVE AFFAIRS

wonder. The essence has the effect of making it much easier
to let go and lay the past to rest, in order to be fully alive
in the present.

Sturt Desert Rose Gossypium sturtianum

Positive: self-esteem.

Negative: guilt, regret, over apologetic.

The Desert Rose essence relates to guilt for things we have done or not done, or feel we should have done or not done. It also relates to the condition of setting excessively high standards for ourselves, which invites comparison with Rock Water (Bach), but whereas Rock Water feels she is living up to the standard set, although perhaps not without a certain effort, Desert Rose feels she is failing miserably.

Very few people grow to adulthood without doing anything to be ashamed of. We learn to be moral through seeing and feeling the consequences of our immoral acts, just as we learn to be careful how we run by scraping our knees. Sometimes we go too far: instead of a scrape the knee receives a deep cut which leaves a scar, and instead of a minor indiscretion we commit some awful deed which keeps us awake years later. Guilt is, however, an entirely useless emotion – if we feel we have done something wrong, we should make what amends are possible and make sure not to do it again so that the lesson is not lost. Repeating an action we know or feel to be wrong is obviously stupid and if we are under some compulsion to do so that is a problem to be solved. Simply feeling guilty about something is a way of opting out of taking responsibility for the necessary action

In Christian theology, despair – the feeling that we have done such wrong that we can never be forgiven or loved – is a sin against the Holy Ghost. This is because it is taught that God always loves, always forgives, and we have no right to refuse that forgiveness. In human terms, our mothers, lovers, children forgive endlessly, and to refuse to forgive ourselves, to persist in the feeling of guilt, is to throw that love and forgiveness back in their faces – it is the worst kind of satanic pride.

The Desert Rose essence helps us not only to see all this with our minds, but to accept it in our bodies, to release our guilt so that we can accept the love and forgiveness of others.

Sundew Drosera spathulata

Positive: grounding, focus.
Negative: disconnectedness.
This is another essence for the sense of being 'not all there'. It has the feel of the personality being divided, and of the vagueness being used as a way of escape. Sundew needs close comparison with the other 'spacey' remedies such as Clematis, White Chestnut (Bach), Arnica (California) and Red Lily (Australian Bush). If the choice is not clear, it may need to be distinguished by muscle test or dowsing.

Sunshine Wattle Acacia terminalis

Positive: optimistic.
Negative: stuck in the past, pessimistic.
This essence is one for the 'dismal Johnnies' who seem to relish anticipating bad luck. If things go swimmingly, they put on a long face and say, 'Of course it won't last'; if things go wrong they say, 'I told you so, what can you expect?' Not only is their glass only half empty, but it is permanently about to fall over! The essence may help them to see that it is possible to look at things in a more optimistic way and that this can even bring about different results.

Tall Yellow Top Senecio magnificus

Positive: sense of 'home'.
Negative: alienation.
This appears to act in a similar way to Sweet Pea (California).

Turkey Bush Calytrix estipulata
Positive: creative expression.
Negative: blocked creativity.
This essence is quite close in character to Iris (California).

Waratah Telopea speciosissima
Positive: faith.
Negative: despair.
Waratah is perhaps one of the most important heart remedies. Ian White feels it is one of the most important remedies of all and has chosen it as the symbol of the Australian Bush Flower Essence project. It is the remedy for suicidal despair, when one feels there is no way out, no future, no hope. There are other remedies for this condition – Sweet Chestnut (Bach) acts almost identically. The homoeopathic Aurum and Ignatia cover aspects of it, Aurum when the loss involved is of wealth and possessions, Ignatia for personal loss, bereavement and separation. When needed, use whichever is most readily available – this is not an occasion for splitting hairs!

Pain comes about from our failure to adapt to change, and this great soul-searing pain comes from our being subjected to enormous changes in our circumstances, so rapidly that we cannot possibly begin to adapt and so we just 'crack up' – our nervous systems come apart under the strain. It is very mysterious exactly how these remedies manage to give us breathing space to catch up and ease the flow of energies to enable us to adapt more fluidly, but that is exactly what they do. From my own experience I know that without question.

We live in a time of great change, on the personal and global level, which means that many more people are going to find themselves in states of crisis. It is most important that we not only find our way through these times but use the challenges and the lessons that they create to advantage, so it is no exaggeration to say that the widespread use of this essence will make a great difference to the future of humanity.

Wedding Bush Ricinocarpus pinifolius

Positive: commitment.
Negative: lack of commitment.
This essence speaks of commitment, whether to a relationship, or to a project or way of life. In relationships, it is valuable for individuals who wish to commit themselves to a long-term relationship, or to couples who wish to strengthen their partnership. In other terms, it is valuable for those who have difficulty in completing projects, and could well be used by business partners in the same way as by couples. Rather than being afraid of being tied down by responsibility, the essence helps us to embrace the opportunity to build gladly and create something worth while.

Wild Potato Bush Solanum quadriloculatum

Positive: able to move.
Negative: weighed down.

Wisteria Wisteria sinensis

Positive: sexual openness.
Negative: frigidity/machismo.
This is an important remedy for sexual problems. The pattern depicted is that of a very Victorian view of a sexual relationship: the woman with her eyes tight shut 'thinking of England' while the man, scarcely bothering to undress, has his rough satisfaction. Although in crude terms the male and female points of view seem to be opposite (the man wanting and 'enjoying' sex, the woman not wanting or enjoying) actually both sides are losing out by failing to

connect the 'sexual act' with anything else – spiritual or emotional contact, or even real physical pleasure. Wisteria is not just about 'sex' but about the quality of relationships that have a sexual component. See also Basil, Hibiscus, Sticky Monkey Flower (California).

Yellow Cowslip Orchid Caladenia flava
Positive: constructive.
Negative: critical.
The last essence in this group is for those who pick and fuss at small details in a way that prevents them achieving a balanced view of a whole picture. They can be very frustrating to work with because they will take up enormous amounts of time and energy over very small points and find it difficult to address broader issues until they are satisfied. In the positive phase, their ability to give attention to detail in a balanced context can be very valuable, so they should be tactfully offered this essence at the first opportunity.

COMBINATION ESSENCES

Ian White has also developed a number of *combination essences* (cf Rescue Remedy) as follows. They are fully described in Ian's book.

- *Radiation essence;* Bush Fuchsia, Crowea, Fringed Violet, Mulla Mulla, Paw Paw, Waratah.
- *Emergency essence:* Fringed Violet, Grey Spider Flower, Sundew, Waratah.
- *Personal power essence:* Dog Rose, Five Corners, Southern Cross, Sturt Desert Rose.
- *Superlearning essence:* Bush Fuchsia, Isopogon, Paw

Paw, Sundew.
* *Vitality:* Banksia, Crowea, Macrocarpa, Old Man Banksia.

8

The Alaskan flower essence project

ORIGINS

The Alaskan flower essences project is largely the work of Steve Johnson. He became interested in the use of the Bach remedies in 1980 and later became involved with the FES. In 1983, he spent time as a fire control officer in the Alaskan wilderness and there began to explore the possibilities of the rich and unique Alaskan flora for making essences. He founded the AFEP to co-ordinate his own work with others studying in the field and was joined by Shabd-sangeet Khalsa, Janice Schofield and Jane Bell. The work has expanded to include the creation of a series of gem elixirs and the environmental essences (see below). Steve's book, *Flower Essences of Alaska*, is required reading for anyone wanting to work with these essences.

Alaska is a vast state containing relatively few people but millions of plants, birds and animals. The northern territory is a place at the extreme limit of the possibilities for human survival, and the other life forms that live there have had to adapt a great deal. Annual plants have the shortest possible season in which to grow and flower, which they do with incredible energy and abundance. Shrubby plants are nearly always dwarfed, hugging the ground for protection against wind and cold. The sunlight falls obliquely through thin clear air. It is obvious that essences made from the flowers of this place will have very special qualities.

THE ESSENCES

The Alaskan essences are divided into three 'kits', which are also subdivided into groups. Generally, the groups comprise plants collected in a single geographical location. The division into kits is partly based on the periods of collection, but also partly on the nature of the remedies. Generally speaking, the essences of Kit 1 are described as the most accessible, those of Kit 3, which includes green flowered and carnivorous plants, as the most subtle, and Kit 2, as you might suppose, somewhere in between. Steve Johnson's book, *Flower Essences of Alaska*, includes details of the collection of the flowers to make the essences, full descriptions of the prescribing pictures, illustrations of the flowers and suitable affirmations to accompany the use of each essence.

PRESCRIBING ALASKAN ESSENCES

As a group, the Alaskan essences seem rather ethereal. The descriptions focus mainly on mental and spiritual ideas which to some may seem rather rarefied and abstract, especially by contrast with the hot-blooded down-to-earth qualities of the Australian Bush remedies. This is quite right: they were born from quiet contemplation in a remote place and they are very strongly connected with those qualities. At the same time, they are created from plants whose lives display great qualities of resourcefulness and inner strength, and these aspects are also brought out in the essences.

Prescribing the Alaskan essences is not complex, but requires perhaps more reflection than some. For anyone interested in working with them I would suggest very careful reading of Steve's book, followed by some meditation on the nature of any essence that seems to have particular appeal. People inclined to working with these essences will have developed a fairly high level of awareness so that self-prescribing accompanied by use of the affirmations and any other supportive measures will quite likely be the best way to work.

THE ALASKAN FLOWER ESSENCES

The essences are listed with brief keynotes to help identify areas of interest, a few points concerning the actual plants, and cross-references to other remedy systems to aid comparison. For full information refer to *Flower Essences of Alaska*.

Alder Alnus Crispa
Keynote: Clarity of perception – Kit 1.

Alpine Azalea Loiseleuria procumbens
Keynote: Unconditional self-acceptance – Kit 2.

The key word here is *unconditional*. A number of essences deal with various aspects of the question of self-acceptance. Rock Water (Bach) which has the idea of only being able to maintain self-regard through a rather grim regime of virtuous acts probably comes closest. Sturt

Desert Rose (Australian Bush) has the sense of being unable to accept the self because of guilt about past events, leading us in turn to consider a condition of Honeysuckle (Bach) which is stuck in the past in a more general way. While Buttercup (California) and Five Corners (Australian Bush) both have the sense of low self-esteem.

This essence addresses in a subtle way the imbalances of energy that come from feeling constrained to behave in a certain way, possibly in accordance with conditioning and against one's natural impulses: 'I can only be a good/ lovable person/feel good about myself as long as I ...' Whereas Desert Rose has (or feels she has) broken this injunction and is therefore not worthy, Alpine Azalea has not and dares not break the unspoken rule, but feels the restriction of impulses which creates deep unease. The essence will act to free this up, making it easier for the person to act in accordance with her real wishes and continue to feel good about herself no matter what.

Balsam Poplar *Populus Balsamifera*
Keynote: Healthy circulation of life energy – Kit 1.

Black Spruce *Picea mariana*
Keynote: Opening to wisdom – Kit 1.

Bladderwort *Utricularia vulgaris*
Keynote: Seeing through illusion – Kit 3.

Blueberry Pollen *Vaccinium uliginosum*
Keynote: Opening to receive – Kit 3.

Blue Elf Viola *Viola sp*
Keynote: Releasing anger through the heart – Kit 1.
States of repressed anger are extremely dangerous as

they cause a blockage of the flow of energy around the heart. This is why chronically angry characters are exceptionally prone to 'angina' and heart disease. The more deeply buried the greater the damage, so an essence like Blue Elf Viola which releases the feeling and the energy from the deepest levels is enormously valuable. Among remedies that will bear comparison, the nearest is probably Sticky Monkeyflower (California). Dagger Hakea (Australian Bush) can also cover a great deal of angry resentment, and is especially appropriate where the anger relates to an identifiable personal hurt. From the Bach series, it is worth drawing comparisons with Holly and Cherry Plum, also not forgetting that anger may be prominent among the distresses covered up by the relentless cheerfulness of an Agrimony.

Bog Blueberry *Vaccinium uliginosum*
Keynote: Welcoming abundance – Kit 2.

Bog Rosemary *Andromeda polifolia*
Keynote: Healing through trust – Kit 2.

Bunchberry *Cornus canadensis*
Keynote: Mental strength and clarity – Kit 2.

Cassandra *Chamaedaphne calyculata*
Keynote: Inner listening – Kit 2.

Cattail Pollen *Typha latifolia*
Keynote: Standing tall in one's truth – Kit 3.

This invites comparison with Mountain Pride (California). The difference is that, whereas Mountain Pride addresses challenges in our truth and integrity that come from outside, e.g. other people's criticisms, Cattail Pollen deals much more with the internal crises of fear and doubt – more like a high potency Elm or Gentian (Bach).

Chiming Bells *Mertensia Paniculata*
Keynote: Experiencing joy in physical existence – Kit 1.

Columbine *Aquilegia formosa*
Keynote: Projecting a strong sense of self – Kit 2.

In our garden, the acquilegia has a great predilection for growing in the middle of paths. It also grows in the borders, but the self-sown 'bandits' are always the best plants by far and I can never bear to cut them down. Although the flowers 'nod' modestly enough they rise on strong, stiff stems, right out of the middle of a perfectly rounded mound of immaculate grey/green foliage – the perfect model of cool, quiet, determined self-possession.

Comandra *Geocauloon lividum*
Keynote: Developing an inner awareness of nature – Kit 3.

Cotton Grass *Eriophorum sp*
Keynote: Moving from pain to healing – Kit 1.

Cow parsnip *Heracleum lanatum*
Keynote: Awareness of inner strength – Kit 2.

This form of cow parsley has all the typical traits of the genus. Its hollow stems grow and branch as widely and stiffly as those of any tree – although herbaceous in nature, it has more the appearance of a woody shrub. Unassuming in the hedgerow, it is endlessly resilient in the face of any amount of mowing or trampling – the qualities which come through in the flower essence.

Dandelion *Taraxacum officinale*
Keynote: Release of emotional tension – Kit 1.

This is, not surprisingly, about identical with the Californian Dandelion.

Fireweed *Epilobium angustifolium*
Keynote: Rejuvenation and renewal – Kit 1.

Forget Me Not *Myosotis Alpestris*
Keynote: Remembering original innocence – Kit 1.

Foxglove *Digitalis Purpurea*
Keynote: Perceptual expansion – Kit 1.

Digitalis is important in allopathic, herbal and homoeopathic medicine for its action on the heart. The flower remedy picture connects this quality with the way that limitation of thought patterns – restricting what we will or will not accept – is a major source of pressure on the heart, and so by opening consciousness to accept different ideas the essence acts indirectly on the same area.

Golden Corydalis *Corydalis aurea*
Keynote: Integration and assimilation – Kit 1.

Grass of Parnassus *Parnassia palustris*
Keynote: Nourishing the body with light – Kit 2.

Green Bells of Ireland *Molucella laevis*
Keynote: Greeting the earth – Kit 1.

Green Bog Orchid *Plantanthera obtusata*
Keynote: Harmonising with the plant kingdom – Kit 3.

Green Fairy Orchid *Hammarbya paludosa*
Keynote: Oneness through inner balance – Kit 3.

Grove Sandwort *Moehringia lateriflora*
Keynote: Strengthening bonds of communication – Kit 2.

Hairy Butterwort *Campanula lasiocarpa*
Keynote: Transition without crisis – Kit 3.

Horsetail *Equisetum arvense*
Keynote: Developing inner communication skills – Kit 2.

The horsetail is a very ancient plant which has been on the planet since before the days of the dinosaurs. It can be thought of, then, as more firmly connected to the earth than most beings and is a remedy of *connection* between different levels of consciousness.

Icelandic Poppy *Papaver icelandica*
Keynote: Spiritual radiance – Kit 1.

Jacob's Ladder *Polemonium pulcherrimum*
Keynote: Spiritual receptivity – Kit 1.

Labrador Tea *Ledum Palustre*
Keynote: Bringing one's life to centre – Kit 1.

The Labrador Tea essence is about bringing energies into balance from a state of transition. Ledum is used in homoeopathy as a wound remedy and it is possible to see how its action in making the transition from the necessary healing state of inflammation and discharge to normality corresponds to the action of flower essence on the mind.

Ladies' Tresses *Spiranthes romanzoffiana*
Keynote: Deep internal alignment – Kit 3.

Lady's Slipper *Cyprepedium guttatum*
Keynote: Focusing and circulating life energy – Kit 1.

It is helpful to compare this closely with the other *Cyprepedium* remedies, Lady's Slipper (California) and Northern Lady's Slipper (Alaska).

Laceflower *Tiarella trifoliata*
Keynote: Self-appreciation – Kit 2.

Lamb's Quarters *Chenopodium album*
Keynote: Balancing the rational and intuitive – Kit 3.

Monkshood *Aconitum delphinifolium*
Keynote: Awareness of one's divine identity – Kit 1.

The *aconites* are beautiful and highly toxic members of the *ranunculus* (buttercup) family. The name derives from the shape of the flower which suggests a friar's cowl. As a homoeopathic remedy it is important for extreme fear which follows from acute trauma, and above all for the fear at the moment of approaching death. The *aconite* patient will be resistant to being touched, as though maintaining separateness was the only hope of avoiding complete dissolution. The flower essence works on a more subtle form of this kind of fear, which leads to an excessive need to separate ourselves from others, again, as though our integrity depended on it, with the result of loneliness and impoverishment.

Moschatel *Adoxa Moschetalina*
Keynote: Developing sensitivity to the plant kingdom – Kit 3.

Mountain Wormwood *Artemisia tilesii*
Keynote: Forgiving old wounds – Kit 2.

Northern Lady's Slipper *Cypripedium passerinum*
Keynote: Reconnecting body and spirit – Kit 3.

Northern Twayblade *Listera borealis*
Keynote: Awareness of light within form – Kit 3.

One-sided Wintergreen *Pyrola secunda*
Keynote: Creating appropriate boundaries – Kit 3.

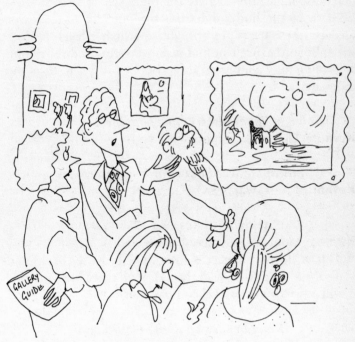

Opium Poppy Papaver sominifera (sic)

Keynote: Integrating activity and rest – Kit 2.

The action of Opium as a drug is well known. In the Nineteenth Century it was popular with artistic types (in the same way as LSD in the 1970s) who found in it both escape from practical stresses of life and stimulation to a flagging imagination. Unfortunately, in this form, it also tends to increase the split between the two sides of the personality – between 'heaven and hell' – as has been documented by writers from Stevenson to Huxley. As a homoeopathic remedy Opium is used for conditions of deep disconnection – where the mind seems disconnected both from the body and from the outside. As a flower essence, these traits are brought to a higher level, healing the split so that we can find it more restful and refreshing to act in a fully connected and grounded way – to be in the moment.

Paper Birch Betula papyrifera

Keynote: Clarity of purpose – Kit 1.

Pineapple Weed Matricaria matricariodes

Keynote: Calm awareness – Kit 2.

Prickly Wild Rose Rosa acicularis

Keynote: Courageous interest in life – Kit 1.

This is closely connected to both Wild Rose (Bach) and California Wild Rose (California). If all three are available it will pay to make careful comparisons.

River Beauty Epilobium latifolium

Keynote: Emotional regeneration and renewal – Kit 2.

Round-leaved Sundew Drosera rotundifolia
Keynote: Surrendering ego attachment – Kit 3.

Shooting Star Dodecathon frigidum
Keynote: Understanding cosmic origins and earthly purpose – Kit 3.

Single Delight Moneses uniflora
Keynote: Healing feelings of isolation – Kit 2.

Sitka Burnet Sanguisorba stipulata
Keynote: Completion on all levels – Kit 3.

Sitka Spruce Pollen Picea sitchensis
Keynote: Timelessness and present action – Kit 3.

Compare with Black Spruce (above) White Spruce (below). The three Spruce remedies are quite closely related, although also quite distinct from each other. They make an interesting set with which to address some far-reaching issues.

Spiraea Spiraea beauverdiana
Keynote: Unconditional acceptance of support – Kit 1.

Sticky Geranium Geranium erianthum
Keynote: Getting unstuck – Kit 2.

Many essences relate to the idea of being 'stuck', indeed, as I wrote many pages ago, the whole idea of flower essence is to 'unstick' something or other. This relates to the same area as Hornbeam (Bach) – that sense of just not being able to get up and get going, of having one's feet stuck in the mud, but on a deeper, more fundamental level. It also has some of the sense of Red Grevillea's (Australian Bush) being stuck in life – of not being able to see the way ahead.

Soapberry Sheperdia Canadensis
Keynote: Harmonising personal and planetary power – Kit 3.

Sphagnum Moss Sphagnum sp
Keynote: Seeing without judgement – Kit 3.

Sunflower Helianthis annula
Keynote: Balancing the masculine – Kit 2.

Sweetgale Myrica gale
Keynote: Releasing core emotional tension – Kit 2.

Sweetgrass Heirochloe odorata
Keynote: Etheric cleansing and completion – Kit 3.

Tamarack Larix laricina
Keynote: Confidence from knowing one's abilities – Kit 2.

This is very closely connected, as an essence, to the Bach Larch. The person needing Tamarack is on the whole more confident and positive than the true Larch, but finds this essence helpful if dealing with temporary challenges tends to knock him 'off centre'.

Tundra Rose Potentilla fruticosa
Keynote: Love of Life – Kit 2.

This pretty shrub is well known in gardens all over the northern hemisphere.

Tundra Twayblade Listera cordata
Keynote: Cellular healing – Kit 3.

Twinflower Linnaea Borealis
Keynote: Clarity of communication – Kit 1.

White Fireweed *Epilobium angustifolium*
Keynote: Deep emotional healing – Kit 3.

White Spruce *Picea glauca*
Keynote: Wisdom and inner balance – Kit 2.

White Violet *Viola renifolia*
Keynote: Opening to divine trust – Kit 2.

Wild Iris *Iris Setosa*
Keynote: Opening to creative potential – Kit 1.

Wild Rhubarb *Polygonum alaskanum*
Keynote: Clearing the channel between heart and mind – Kit 3.

Willow *Salix bebbiana*
Keynote: Mental flexibility and resilience – Kit 1.

Yarrow *Achillea borealis*
Keynote: Strengthening one's inner light – Kit 1.

Yellow Dryas *Dryas drummondii*
Keynote: Strength of identity and individuality – Kit 2.

9

Exotic and indigenous

The development of new flower remedies seems to have acquired an unstoppable momentum. In addition to the groups described in previous chapters, there are many that are so far less well known but may in the future come to be equally or even more important. It would take a far larger book than this to cover all the available essences in any sort of detail, but this chapter gives brief descriptions of some groups that may well be worth following up. I begin with sets of remedies which have been developed in Britain since Dr Bach's time, going on to look at some from more exotic locations.

THE BAILEY FLOWER ESSENCES

Origins

The Bailey flower essences are the work of Arthur Bailey PhD, a former senior lecturer in Electronic and Electrical Engineering at the University of Bradford. Bailey began investigating dowsing out of scientific curiosity and was alarmed as well as intrigued to find that it worked! He is a former president and scientific adviser to the British Society of Dowsers. He began using the Bach remedies and developed some skill in selecting them by dowsing, which led him to wonder whether the dowsing method might be used to discover other healing plants. He duly discovered a number of new remedies both by dowsing and through direct intuition. An initial group of six has steadily expanded to around 45. Because the remedies were discovered by dowsing, it took some time for their precise healing properties to be established. This was mainly done through selecting remedies for patients by dowsing and building up the remedy pictures from the patients they had helped. Dr Bailey originally developed the essences for his own use and interest but was persuaded to make them available by persistent requests from other practitioners. He has produced a small handbook describing the remedies, as well as *Dowsing for Health*, a general account of clinical dowsing, and plans to produce a more complete work on the essences and their preparation.

The essences

Most of the Bailey essences are made from flowers, although a few use other parts of the respective plants. Most are made by the sun method of infusion in water: for the materials that are resistant to this method he has used infusion in alcohol, which he finds more satisfactory than boiling. Quite a number of the remedies are made from plant sources which are used in other essences or in homoeopathy. The descriptions of these essences do not generally correspond to their counterparts, and I am at a loss to know which aspect of the air or soil or Yorkshire would account for such extreme differences.

Prescribing the Bailey essences

Dr Bailey states that the Bailey essences are compatible with and complementary to the Bach remedies, so that the two groups can be freely used together. Many of the pictures resemble those of the Bach series, but with a more detailed focus, as it were, zooming up on some detail of one of the Bach pictures. He personally prefers to prescribe by dowsing, but the remedies are well enough described for the interview method to be quite successful for an experienced user. Dr Bailey's book, *The Bailey Flower Essences*, is absolutely essential for anyone working with these essences. The 'keynotes' below are my inadequate paraphrases of Dr Bailey's eloquent descriptions. The accompanying notes concentrate on points of comparison within the group and with others.

Bistort Polygonum bistorta
Keynote: protection in change.

This essence appears to cover the same area as Walnut (Bach) but with more intensity. It is especially adapted to changes which give rise to great pain and anxiety.

Blackthorn Prunus Spinosa
Keynote: despair.
Close to Sweet Chestnut, but particularly suited to the Rock Water type.

Bluebell Hyacinthoides non scripta
Keynote: self-love, self-respect.

Bog Asphodel Narthecium ossifragum
Keynote: the willing slave: balancing one's own needs with others'.

This is a complex essence: compared to the Bach remedies it covers aspects of Centaury, Vervain and Rock Water. An important remedy for therapists and any who may fall into the trap of 'do-gooding'.

Bracken Pteridium aquilinum *(alcoholic extract)*
Keynote: adult children: dependency.

Bracken Pteridium aquilinum *(aqueous extract)*
Keynote: acceptance of suppressed intuitive nature.

Butterbur Petasites hybridus
Keynote: acceptance of personal power.

Buttercup Ranunculus Acris
Keynote: cynicism.

Ranunculus Acris is used in homoeopathy. Although attractive, the field buttercup is extremely bitter and indeed poisonous. The character of the essence resembles those saloon bar types who are always able to raise a laugh by disparaging someone else, not that they have ever done anything particularly worthy themselves. If we compare this one to the Bach Beech, we find that Beech, although rather negative in approach, at least sometimes criticises from honest motives: Buttercup addresses that streak of plain nastiness that is not too far from the surface in rather too many of us. As with all unpleasant behaviour, the perpetrator is the first and worst victim – which does not make the habit any easier to break. In fact, the Buttercup type is rather in the position of Mephistopheles, in despairing (wrongly) of his own salvation and being determined to drag as many others into damnation with him as possible – not in the hope of any joy, but because misery, as they say, loves company. It can be dangerous to get too close to these people, since there can be a sort of fascination, but if you risk it, perhaps a drop or two in his beer ...?

Charlock Sinapis Arvensis
Keynote: growing up – taking responsibility.

This is made from the identical plant to Dr Bach's

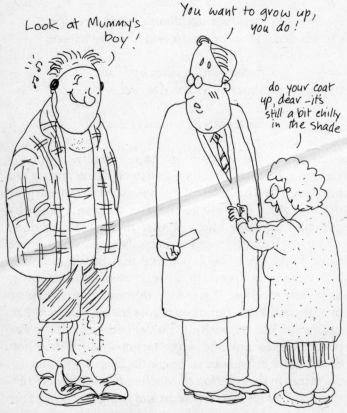

CHARLOCK – REFUSING TO GROW UP IN A PETER PAN SORT OF WAY AND AQUEOUS BRACKEN WHERE THE STATE OF PROLONGED CHILDHOOD IS ENFORCED BY A PARENT ...

Mustard, yet it comes with a radically different description which defies the attempt to make a lucid connection, except that the inarticulate gloom of Mustard could be seen as a childish trait. The important distinction within this group is between Charlock, refusing to grow up in a Peter Pan sort of way, and Aqueous Bracken where the state of prolonged childhood is enforced by a parent who will not allow their child to grow up. The one irresponsible, the other deprived.

Double Snowdrop Galanthus nivalis 'flore plena'
Keynote: eases rigid, authoritarian attitudes.

Early Purple Orchid Orchis Mascula
Keynote: unblocking: keeping change going.
Since moving energy and promoting change is what the flower remedies are all about, this can possibly be seen as a 'master essence' within this group, in the same way as Lotus in the Himalayan essences (see below).

Firethorn Pyracantha atlantioides
Keynote: balancing energies: stability.

Flowering Currant Ribes Sanguineum
Keynote: giving up – keeping going.
This occupies similar ground to the Bach Gorse, but perhaps depicts a more extreme condition, verging on that of Sweet Chestnut.

Foxglove Digitalis Purpurea
Keynote: confusion – direction.
The description of this essence relates very loosely to the description in the California series and to the homoeo-

pathic picture. It describes in a different way difficulties in the relationship between heart and head.

Hairy Sedge *Carex Hirta*
Keynote: poor memory: indifference.

We tend to use memory selectively, remembering things we like and 'conveniently' forgetting things we dislike, or do not want to be bothered with. In childhood, this game, like many, can be played without much harm, but as we get older and use it more it tends to take us over. The loss of memory in later life is strongly associated with rigid attitudes and beliefs, since ignoring and forgetting contrary evidence is the easiest way to defend a view that has no rational foundation. In association with other essences, and for willing patients, this may well hold the key to arresting and preventing mental deterioration in later life.

Honesty *Lunaria Annua*
Keynote: honesty (honestly!).

Leopardsbane *Doronicum paradalianches*
Keynote: coping with awakening perceptions.

Lesser Stitchwort *Stellaria graminea*
Keynote: a new essence released in 1994, Dr Bailey describes it thus: 'For "possession", i.e. for those whose behaviour is dominated by strongly held ideas or by other beings'.'

Lilac *Syringa vulgaris 'Massena'*
Keynote: lack of growth.
Compare with Almond (California).

EXOTIC AND INDIGENOUS 169

Lily of the Valley *Convallaria Majalis*
Keynote: another new one in 1994: 'For yearning. For those who have become blocked by desiring the unattainable' (Bailey Flower Essences newsletter).

Marigold *Calendula officinalis*
Keynote: materialism, scepticism.

The particular focus to this essence is the 'scoffer' at anything not immediately understood or verifiable as 'scientific fact'. The description given fits the same personality as the identical Calendula (California) in its hardness and sharpness, and in the sense that this aggressive front is used as a defence from fear of what a more open response might bring.

Marsh Thistle *Cirsium palustre*
Keynote: locked in the past – accepting change.

Not in the Honeysuckle (Bach) sense of nostalgic longing for the past, but for the insistence on bringing the past into the present – living 'the way we have always lived', stuck in the hamster wheel of fixed routines out of habit and fear of the future.

Milk Thistle *Sonchus oleraceus*
Keynote: opening the heart.

Monkshood *Aconitum Napellus*
Keynote: objectivity concerning the past.

Compare with Monkshood (Alaska). This plant is another of the great stalwarts of homoeopathy and a close relative of the Alaskan Monkshood. The description of this essence is at first sight very different from those which occur in the other sources, although with more thought a relationship is visible. The homoeopathic Aconite is a very fearful remedy, which frequently occurs in childhood illness. An event which is strongly felt as a child frequently takes on an unreal, out of proportion appearance, and the same happens to the feelings which are embedded at that time. This essence is said to help in letting go of the exaggerated fears and feelings attached to childhood events (possibly even those where Aconite should have been given at the time) creating freedom and understanding in the adult.

Moss *Discranella heteromalla*
Keynote: fear of the darkness within.

Nasturtium *Tropaeolum majus*
Keynote: initiating change.

In this series, the Nasturtium essence is associated with overcoming negative feelings associated with change. The resemblance to the Californian essence from the same plant is not obvious, yet the fear of change can be seen as related to the imbalance between emotion and intellect described in the Californian form: the intellect likes to be in control and is therefore mistrustful of change because change involves a period of not knowing. Although we like to think of intellect as an enabler, when it gets out of hand its influence is deadening (as in the case of 'scientists' who refuse to accept that flower essences work, even though they see their effects) and this is what the Nasturtium essence helps to overcome.

Oxalis *Oxalis ptychoclada*
Keynote: throat (literal and metaphorical).

Pine Cones *Pinus sylvestris*

Keynote: trapped, dependent on authority – independence.

This has an interesting relationship to the Bach Pine since the dependency and inadequacy which leads one to surrender to (sometimes dubious) authority figures is based in a feeling of guilt and unworthiness. The Cone remedy, then, expresses the flower picture, but in a more focused and concentrated way.

Pink Purslane *Montia siberica*

Keynote: open mind.

Compare with Bauhinia (Australian Bush).

Red Clover *Trifolium pratense*

Keynote: emotional block: right/left brain balance.

Rhododendron *Rhododendron ponticum*

Keynote: 'headbangers'.

Those who will spend all day pushing when the sign on the door says 'pull'.

Scarlet Pimpernel *Anargallis arvensis*

Keynote: obsession/possession – freedom.

Siberian Spruce *Picea omorica*

Keynote: assertiveness.

Single Snowdrop *Galanthus nivalis*

Keynote: breaking through.

Soapwort *Saponaria ocymoides*

Keynote: confusion.

Solomon's Seal *Polygonatum verticillatum*
Keynote: busy mind.

This compares to a mixture of White Chestnut and Vervain: the mind always cluttered and much rushing and striving with little effect. The essence is said to help one learn to achieve more, quietly.

Spring Squill *Scilla verna*
Keynote: loneliness from breaking free.

Sumach *Rhus typhina*
Keynote: accepting one's potential.

Thrift *Armeria maritima*
Keynote: earthing psychic abilities.

Tufted Vetch *Vicia cracca*
Keynote: clarifying sexual self-image.

Valerian *Valeriana officinalis*
Keynote: 'lost child'.

Welsh Poppy *Meconopsis cambrica*
Keynote: loss of inspiration/'bewitched' – regaining the path.

Witch Hazel *Hamamelis mollis*
Keynote: pleasing others – centring in the self.
  Compare with Rock Water (Bach).

Wood Anemone *Anemone nemorosa*
Keynote: karmic problems.
  See also the Karmic essences on pages 188–89.

Yew *Taxus baccata*

Keynote: releasing rigidity.

Compare with Bauhinia (Australian Bush).

There are also three composite Bailey remedies:

GRIEF

- **Sheep's Sorrel** *Rumex acetocella*.
- **Dog Rose** *Rosa Canina*.
- **Yorkshire Fog** *Holcus Lanathus*.
- **Trailing Saint John's Wort** *Hypericum humifusum*.

TRANQUILLITY

- **Heath Bedstraw** *Galium saxatile*.
- **Tree Mallow** *Lavatera Arborea*.
- **Fuji Cherry** *Prunus incisa*.

OBSESSION

- **Ragwort**
- **Indian Balsam**
- **Field Woundwort**

This new (1994) remedy is described in the *Bailey Flower Essences Journal* no 1. Traditionally, one would associate obsessive thoughts with the Bach White Chestnut, but Honeysuckle, Holly, Cherry Plum are all in there too, addressing different aspects or shades of feeling. Dr Bailey's article deals especially with the need to deal with the disconcerting effect of suddenly finding the mind emptied, which can make one want to 'turn the noise up' all over again. Many users of White Chestnut find that, although the remedy works, the mind finds it hard to give up its habits so that the relief is temporary unless one is prepared to really work consciously at changing the thought patterns. While permanent change will always require some work this interesting new essence may make it just a little easier.

GREEN MAN ESSENCES (SIMON LILLEY)

Simon Lilley is another 'English Independent', following Dr Bach in producing essences according to his own intuition. His tree essences cover 74 trees grown in the British Isles and offer separate 'male' and 'female' forms where the trees are 'sexed'. Many of the tree essences are from the same species as remedies of the Bach series. However, except in the case of Elm, the descriptions vary widely.

Green Man also produce a series of 26 flower essences from herbaceous plants. A number of these overlap with the California and Bailey groups, others are unique to this series.

Some of these essences do not as yet have descriptions and keys: they cannot therefore be prescribed by the interview method, but need to be selected by kinesiology, dowsing or intuitive methods.

All the essences can be supplied in the usual tincture form, in non-alcoholic preparation, or in homoeopathic potency to order. Green Man essences have a high reputation for quality and effectiveness among professional practitioners. The keywords accompanying the listing are Simon's. He will be glad to give further information.

- *Alder*: 'release'.
- *Apple*: 'detoxification'.
- *Ash*: 'strength'.
- *Bay*: 'energy'.
- *Beech*: 'easy going'.

- *Bird Cherry*: 'sensuality'.
- *Black Poplar*: 'solidity'.
- *Blackthorn*: 'circulation'.
- *Birch*: 'beauty'.
- *Box*: 'clarity'.
- *Catalpa*: 'joy'.
- *Cherry Laurel*: 'balance of mind.'.
- *Cherry Plum*: 'confidence'.
- *Copper Beech*: 'depression'.
- *Crack Willow*: 'spiritual sun'.
- *Elder*: 'self-worth'.
- *Elm*: 'enthusiasm'.
- *Field Maple*: 'aching heart'.
- *Gean, Wild Cherry*: 'soothing'.
- *Giant Redwood*: 'weight of responsibility'.
- *Glastonbury Thorn*: 'out of the woods'.
- *Gorse*: 'integration'.
- *Great Sallow*: 'soul'.
- *Hawthorn*: 'love'.
- *Hazel*: 'skills'.
- *Holly*: 'power of peace'.
- *Holm Oak*: 'negative emotions'.
- *Hornbeam*: 'right action'.
- *Italian Alder*: 'protected peace'.
- *Ivy*: 'fear'.
- *Judas Tree*: 'channelling'.
- *Laburnum*: 'detoxification'.
- *Larch*: 'will to express'.
- *Lawson Cypress*: 'the Path'.
- *Leyland Cypress*: 'freedom'.
- *Lilac*: 'spine'.
- *Lucombe Oak*: 'creative energy'.
- *Magnolia*: 'restlessness'.
- *Manna Ash*: 'happy with oneself'.

- *Mimosa*: 'sensitivity'.
- *Monterey Pine*: 'connectedness'.
- *Norway Maple*: 'healing love'.
- *Oak*: 'manifestation'.
- *Pear*: 'serenity'.
- *Persian Ironwood*: 'alienation'.
- *Pine*: 'insight'.
- *Pittespora*: 'in two minds'.
- *Plane*: 'fine judgement'.
- *Plum*: 'empowerment'.
- *Privet*: 'old wounds'.
- *Red Chestnut*: 'fear for others'.
- *Red Oak*: 'practical support'.
- *Rowan*: 'nature'.
- *Silver Maple*: 'moods'.
- *Spindle*: 'self-integration'.
- *Stag's Horn Sumach*: 'meditation'.
- *Strawberry Tree*: 'quietude'.
- *Sweet Chestnut*: 'the now'.
- *Sycamore*: 'lightening up'.
- *Tamarisk*: 'fire of transformation'.
- *Tree Lichen*: 'wisdom'.
- *Tree of Heaven*: 'heaven on earth'.
- *Tulip Tree*: 'spiritual nourishment'.
- *Viburnum*: 'reassurance'.
- *Weeping Willow*: 'ego'.
- *White Poplar*: 'starting again'.
- *White Willow*: 'true self'.
- *Whitebeam*: 'fairies'.
- *Yellow Buckeye*: 'devas'.
- *Yew*: 'protection'.

CRYSTAL HERBS (SHIMARA) ESSENCES

Shimara is another channel of 'John', the source of many of the California essences (see chapter 6). The essences produced by Crystal Herbs in England are, however, not clones of the California series; although many of them are similar there are others that are unique, or bear different descriptions.

The similarity is strong enough, nonetheless, for me not to include a detailed listing here: Crystal Herbs and their London outlet, Yantra, produce a detailed catalogue.

PERELANDRA VIRGINIAN FLOWER ESSENCES

The Virginian essences from the Eastern Seaboard are another large group of American essences, broadly similar in nature and scope to the California set. The essences, and relevant books and information, are available in the UK from the FGRA. Space does not permit detailed description or comparison with other groups here.

HIMALAYAN TREE AND FLOWER ESSENCES

There is currently great interest in essences from the flowers of tropical, subtropical and equatorial regions. The first such group to achieve widespread notice is the Himalayan essences. They form a unique group of essences with only a few botanical overlaps with other groups. Some of the remedy characters are quite unique – others overlap more or less with the Australian and Californian essences in particular. As one might expect, they are focused equally on the divine and the profane, with a great emphasis on humanising and centering the emotions and spiritual desires in the body. They are listed here with brief

keynotes for reference, and indications for comparisons
with other remedies.

Ashoka Tree
Keynote: sorrow into joy.
  Compare with Waratah (Australian Bush), Bleeding
Heart (California).

Bougainvillaea
Keynote: connection with higher purpose.

Cannon Ball Tree (female)
Keynote: negativity towards sex.
  Compare with Alpine Lily (California).

Christ's Thorn
Keynote: redemption from guilt.
  Compare with Sturt Desert Rose (Australian Bush).

Day Blooming Jessamine
Keynote: redemption through suffering.
  Compare Penstemon (California).

Indian Mulberry
Keynote: group hatred – reconciliation.

Ixora
Keynote: revitalising relationships.
  Compare Wedding Bush (Australian Bush).

Lotus
Keynote: Clearing mind – the master essence.

Malabar Nut Tree
Keynote: feeling of superiority/prejudice – integration.

Neem
Keynote: excessive mentalisation – centering in the heart.

Nilgiri Longy Plant
Keynote: humanises relations between teachers and students.

Pagoda Tree
Keynote: integrating sex and love.
   Compare with Hibiscus (California), Wisteria (Australian Bush).

Parval
Keynote: religious fanaticism – openness of heart.
   Compare with Rock Water (Bach).

Peacock Flower
Keynote: rehabilitation.

Pill Bearing Spurge
Keynote: accident prone – resentment.

Red Hibiscus
Keynote: emotional warmth.

Red Silk Cotton Tree
Keynote: spiritual purity – avoids false gurus.

Rippy Hillox Plant
Keynote: negativity about sex.

Slow Match Tree
Keynote: healing relationships.

Swallow Wart
Keynote: subconscious disharmony.

Tassel Flower
Keynote: forgiveness in family distress.
Compare with Dagger Hakea (Australia Bush).

Teak Wood Tree
Keynote: refreshes mind in old age.

Torroyia Roshi Plant
Keynote: environmental awareness.

Water Lily
Keynote: sensuality.

White Coral Tree
Keynote: narrow mindedness.
Compare with Slender Rice Flower (California).

Yellow Silk Cotton Tree
Keynote: freeing from the desire for power.

AMAZON ORCHID ESSENCES AND HAWAIIAN ENDEMIC ESSENCES

The Amazon orchid essences are made from rare epiphytic orchids which live high up in the tree canopy above the Amazon rainforest. The Hawaiian endemic essences are made from flowers unique to the Hawaiian islands. Both of these groups are relatively new and information on them is somewhat sparse at the time of writing. They can be obtained in the UK from the FGES who will also be best able to give information on these and other new developments.

10

Beyond the fringe

As described at the beginning of this book, the flower essences come under the general heading of vibrational medicine. The vibrational principle has recently been applied to creating essences from non-plant sources, as described below. These obviously represent one of the farther regions of 'natural healing', and there may be some for whom all this sort of thing strains credulity too far. To anyone having that difficulty, I can only say that 15 years ago I would not have countenanced any of this stuff for a moment, liking to think of myself as a supremely rational being and extremely resistant to anything at all 'flakey'. One experience having led to another, I no longer feel the same certainty about what is and what is not. I have seen so many extraordinary things happen which defeat 'scientific' reduction that my first reaction to a new idea these days is always, 'why not?' Beyond that I never 'believe' nor disbelieve: I simply like to observe results – and I have seen many very interesting results from the unlikeliest practices. So, the descriptions of the essences which follow here are presented for what they are worth, based on the source information, not to be 'believed' or not, but to be tried and used, or not, as interest dictates. The accounts given of the theoretical bases of these techniques are in accordance with the thinking of those who practise them, and may not correspond to accepted 'scientific' thought.

LIGHT ESSENCES

The use of light and colour as tools of healing is very well established. As I observed in the introductory chapter, all matter is energy and all life originates from light energy, so it is not surprising that this should be so. Bathing the body or just the eyes with light is a well-known and effective therapy, and a number of techniques have been developed which use the individual ray frequencies of the different colours for specific healing purposes. There is broad agreement among colour healers of all backgrounds about the significance and effect of the different colours, which leaves the question of the most effective way of making these energies available.

Techniques used include:

- Bathing the body in coloured light while naked or dressed in light, white clothes.
- Taking coloured light directly into the eyes.
- Exposing the body to sunlight while dressed in coloured clothing (especially silk) which acts as a filter.
- Using sunlight and coloured filters to energise water or other liquids – making essences.

Although the other techniques are effective, they also have practical limitations. All the reasons given in chapter 1 for the use of essences in general as a mode of treatment apply very strongly to light essences: using water as a carrier is arguably the safest and most effective way of assimilating any form of energy into the system, and the convenience of having a rainbow in a bottle (or, at least, a small collection of bottles) cannot be denied.

Light essences are prepared by Simon Lilley (Green Man essences) and a few other suppliers. Simon offers a specialised service of creating mixed light essences for a particular situation by postal or telephone consultation.

For those who would like to make their own light essences, Hygiea Studios supply hand-blown full-spectrum filter glass in the spectrum colours. The appropriate colour should be placed on top of a container of water in full sunlight for a few hours. It is also possible to use commercial plastic colour filters such as those made by Strand Lighting which are available in a wide range of colours, including the pure spectrum shades.

The basic colours with their assignments are:

- *Magenta*: change.
- *Red*: energy.
- *Orange*: joy.
- *Yellow*: clarity, discrimination.
- *Green*: balance, calm.
- *Blue*: immunity, communication.
- *Indigo*: relaxation, perception.
- *Violet*: dignity, release of full potential.
- *Pink*: love.
- *White*: transformation.
- *Ultra-violet*: cosmic connections.

Amplification of these ideas and the uses of these energies can be found in any text on colour healing. A few are suggested in the bibliography.

Crystal and gem elixirs

Crystal (gem) healing takes the basic argument underlying light and colour healing a step further. Gemstones are extremely dense minerals formed by unique forces of heat and pressure: in other words they are, in effect, patterns of energy made solid. They are also translucent and of particular colours, so that light which passes through a gem acquires the general energy pattern proper to the colour – 'flavoured', as it were, by the particular structural energy pattern of the stone.

In my earlier life, crystal healing was one of the ideas for which I reserved a special degree of cynicism and scorn. Later on I encountered the force of a healing gemstone, and learned to respect the craft of working with crystals as much as any other.

A gem essence, or 'elixir', can be prepared in the same way as an ordinary light essence, and the arguments for doing so are, if anything, stronger, since while colour filters can be reliably manufactured at minimal cost, gemstones of exceptional quality are rare, costly – and impossible to duplicate. By using the essence mode for transmitting their energy, the power of rare and wonderful gems can be made much more widely available than by any other means.

The possibly tricky area is the validation of the properties of individual gems or essences, and here there is still a great deal of room for charlatanism as well as the real thing. Kinesiology, dowsing, intuition and channelling of information have all made contributions to the basic 'data bank' concerning the gems that are used, and this is reinforced by user feedback from practitioners and patients.

A number of suppliers are dealing in gem essences. I strongly suggest dealing only with the most reputable, or with people of whom you have personal knowledge. Ask for as much information as possible about the gem sources used and, if in any doubt, ask a reliable kinesiologist or dowser to help you check the quality and suitability of the essence.

The Flower and Gem Essence Society have a range of 216 gem and crystal essences, of which 96 are supplied in kits (of 24 each). Yantra offer a range of 160 or so. The essences supplied in the FGES kits are regarded as having well-established characters and purposes; others are classed as research essences, to be prescribed intuitively and results reported.

ENVIRONMENTAL ESSENCES

The Alaskan environmental essences, which come from the same source as the Alaskan flowers, are the first attempt to embody raw natural forces in the form of an essence. No doubt others are on the way. As I said in the introduction, all the energies embodied in essences of any kind are basically electromagnetic and act on the body through its electromagnetic fields. The idea of embodying elemental forces in the form of essences may seem strange at first, but is really no different in principle from the creation of light essences. The main difficulty is finding a location where the energies are accessible without distortion. This would suggest somewhere without large concentrations of artificial light, or indeed electricity supplies; where the atmosphere is clear and free from polluting smogs; and close to natural energy centres of the earth.

Alaska suggests itself since, as well as meeting all the general criteria, it is very close to the magnetic north pole, the greatest concentration of electromagnetic energy on this planet. It also straddles the Arctic circle. This gives special force to the solar energies, since the transition from night to day takes place only every six months, at the equinoxes.

The environmental essences were prepared by placing bowls of pure water on the ground, exposed to the atmosphere and sunlight, for a long enough period to become attuned to the natural vibrations. The 'ice essences' were prepared using meltwater from the locations. Through the action of the forces present at the particular place and time, they embody particular interactions of the four elements: fire, earth, air and water. The characters assigned to the essences are based on the intuitions which arose at the time of their making.

The Alaskan environmental essences

- Northern Lights
- Polar Ice
- Portage Glacier
- Rainbow Glacier
- Solstice Storm
- Solstice Sun

CHAKRA ESSENCES

The chakras of Indian medicine are energy centres in the subtle body which correspond loosely to major plexuses in the nerve system of the physical body. The essences, which are produced by Yantra in London, correspond to the seven major chakras of tradition:

- Crown (pineal)
- Brow (pituitary)

- Throat
- Heart
- Solar plexus
- Sacral
- Base (genital)

In Indian medicine, health is maintained to be largely a matter of balancing the energies at these critical points. The channelling of these energies into remedies seems to bring the idea of healing essences full circle – using the body's energies directly to rebalance others. The Yantra catalogue states: 'These vibrations have been channelled into the bottle directly from source, via the raymasters and angels, with love, for the healing of mankind.'

KARMIC ESSENCES

The Bach remedies deal very much with present and recent emotions. Various of the 'new remedies', e.g. the Alaskans and certain of the Californians, aspire to deal with the 'realms of higher consciousness' and with the relations between the physical and subtle bodies. The karmic essences from Yantra are a special group of flower essences, claimed to 'vibrate on a higher level' and to deal with emotional problems derived from our karma, understood as the burden of experience of our past lives which forms the basis of lessons we have to learn in the present one. People who feel strongly that their present difficulties may have a karmic basis will find this group of essences particularly interesting. Seven essences are described in this class, together with a 'trinity' of spiritual essences which are said to form a bridge between the 'ordinary', emotionally based essences and this more rarefied group. The dosage for these remedies is four drops, four times a day:

the karmic essences should be taken in this way for only three days at a time.

THE SEVEN KARMIC ESSENCES

- *White Bluebell*: over-sensitivity.
- *Pink Rose*: fear.
- *Wild Iris*: over-care and concern for others.
- *Wild Orchid*: uncertainty.
- *Water Lily*: loneliness.
- *Valerian*: disinterest.
- *Yellow Rattle*: despair and despondency.

THE TRINITY

- *Geranium*: darkness into light.
- *Fuchsia*: unblocking energy – heart chakra.
- *Lily*: comfort – serenity.

In conclusion

The interest in and use of flower remedies and related vibrational essences will clearly continue to grow, possibly at an even faster rate than hitherto. In the process, as in any growth activity, many seeds will be sown, not all of which will survive into healthy plants, or bear fruit. Time alone will tell which groups of remedies, new or old, will play the most important parts. It may be that some will be of universal value; or that all will be found to be more useful to some than to others – and even that some of those currently appearing may not be all they seem. This will become clear through many people using the essences and collecting and sharing their experiences. If you have read this far you are probably either already practising with essences or strongly drawn to this way of working. I hope that this book has been, and will continue to be, useful to you as a guide to your explorations, and that they will bring you health, understanding and happiness.

Useful addresses

The Dr Edward Bach Centre
Mount Vernon
Sotwell
Wallingford
Oxon OX10 0PZ

Bailey Flower Essences
Yorkshire indigenous essences
Dr A R Bailey
7/8 Nelson Road
Ilkley
W Yorks LS29 8HN
Tel: 0943 602177
Fax: 0943 817706

Flower and Gem Remedy Association
The Flower and Gem Remedy Association
Suite 1
Castle Farm
Clifton Road
Deddington
Oxon OX15 0TP
Tel: 0869 37349
Fax: 0869 37376

Main UK suppliers for most of the 'foreign' flower essences. Also runs workshops and supplies: essential oils, colour remedies, herbal treatments, creams, lotions, books, courses.

Green Man Essences
Simon Lilley
2 Kerswell Cottages
Exminster
Exeter
Devon EX6 8AY
Tel: 0392 832005
Tree essences, flower essences, light essences.

Healing Herbs
Julian & Martine Barnard
PO Box 65
Hereford
Tel: 0873 890218
Fax: 0873 890314

Noma (Complex Homoeopathy) Ltd
Sylvia A Austen, MD
Unit 3
1–16 Hollybrook Road
off Winchester Road
Upper Shirley
Southampton SO1 6RB
Tel: 0703 770513
Fax: 0703 702459
Pacific flower essences, also essential oils.

Yantra at Strange Attractions
204 Kensington Park Road
London W11 1NR

Tel: 071 229 9646
Fax: 071 229 4781
Importers of Himalayan essences. Main suppliers of crystal herbs, essences.

USA

Flower Essence Repertory
Kaminski, P and Katz, R
The Flower Essence Society
Nevada City
USA 91631306 0 9

The repertory covers the Bach Remedies as well as the FES Californians. The descriptions of the Californian essences are excellent, and those of the Bach Remedies perfectly sound. The repertory section is not as complete as it might be: quite a few rubrics are entirely missing, but it is a useful tool and the only attempt at the task made so far.

Alaskan Flower Essence Project
Alaskan Flower Essences
PO Box 1369
Homer
Alaska 99603–1369
907 235 2188

Flower Essence Society
PO Box 459
Nevada City
California 95959
Tel: 1 916 265 9163
Fax: 1 916 265 6467
Flower Essence Repertory, primary source for California essences and gem elixirs.

AUSTRALIA

The Australian Flower Remedy Society
PO Box 531
Spit Junction
NSW 2088
Australia
Tel: 0869 37349
Fax: 0869 37376

Australian bush flower essences. Publishes a quarterly
newsletter and runs workshops. Membership 20 Aus.
dollars.

FURTHER READING

Heal Thyself
Bach, Edward
C.W. Daniel & Co. Saffron Walden, Essex.
Dr Bach's first book deals, not with flower remedies as
such, but with his general philosophy of sickness and
healing.

The Twelve Healers and Other Remedies
Bach, Edward
C.W. Daniels & Co. Saffron Walden, Essex.
The essential original description of the Bach Remedies.

A Guide to the Bach Flower Remedies
Barnard, Julian
C.W. Daniels & Co. Saffron Walden, Essex.
A valuable guide by an outstanding practitioner and
leading maker of remedies.

Patterns of Life Force
Barnard, Julian
Flower Remedy Programme
An exploration of the underlying principles of how the remedies work.

Collected Writings of Dr Bach
Barnard, Julian (ed)
Ashgrove Press
A collection of Dr Bach's early writings, unpublished elsewhere.

The Healing Herbs of Dr Bach
Barnard, Julian & Martine
Ashgrove Press
A definitive text on the preparation and use of Dr Bach's remedies.

Handbook of the Bach Flower Remedies
Chancellor, Philip M
C.W. Daniels & Co. Saffron Walden, Essex.
A worthy attempt at a comprehensive guide: the descriptions are amplified with numerous case histories which make good points, but one has to be careful not to regard the anecdotal case as defining the essence. Beautifully produced and illustrated.

Bach Flower Remedies for Women
Howard, Judy
C.W. Daniels & Co. Saffron Walden, Essex.

The Bach Flower Remedies Step by Step
Howard, Judy
C.W. Daniels & Co. Saffron Walden, Essex.
A very handy practical prescriber.

The Story of Mount Vernon
Howard, Judy
C.W. Daniels & Co. Saffron Walden, Essex.
An informative history of Dr Bach's work and the work of
the Bach centre up to the present.

Dictionary of The Bach Flower Remedies
Hyne-Jones, T.W.
C.W. Daniels & Co. Saffron Walden, Essex.
Concise reference to positive and negative aspects.

Questions and Answers on the Bach Flower Remedies
Ramsell, John
The Bach Centre, Mount Vernon, Sotwell, Oxon.
This useful little handbook clarifies a number of issues
concerning the use of the remedies and also sets out the
Bach Centre 'party line' on a number of matters.

Bach Flower Therapy Theory and Practice
Scheffer, Mechthild
Thorsons Ltd. Northants, England.
The most original and insightful writing on the remedies
since Dr Bach's own books. Recommended.

The Bach Remedies Repertory
Wheeler, F.J.
C.W. Daniels & Co. Saffron Walden, Essex.
A well-thought-out repertory which presents all the remedies connected to a particular expression, to aid comparison and selection. Very valuable as an aid to the study of
the remedies.

Flower Remedies Natural Healing with Flower Essences
Wildwood, Christine
Element Books Ltd, Shaftesbury, Dorset.

The Bach Flower Remedies Illustrations and Preparations
Weeks, N and Bullen, V
C.W. Daniels & Co. Saffron Walden, Essex.
This book is entirely devoted to the plants and their preparation for those who are interested: it does not contain any information on the use of the remedies. Illustrated with good photographs.

Flower Essences of Alaska
Johnson, Steve M.
Alaskan Flower Essence Project, Homer, Alaska.
The original description of this very interesting group: essential!

Bush Flower Essences
White, Ian
Findhorn Press, Forres, Scotland.
The definitive text on this subject.

Handbook of The Bailey Flower Essences
Bailey, Arthur
Ilkley Healing Centre, Ilkley, Yorks.
Original descriptions of these new remedies, and of Dr Bailey's prescribing method. Available only from Ilkley by post. A more comprehensive book is in preparation.

Flower Essences and Vibrational Healing
Gurudas
Cassandra Press, PO Box 868, San Rafael CA 94915, USA.
The primary source of information, both on the actual remedies and on their esoteric origins. The essences are divided into those which act primarily on the physical system (mostly plants known in the herbal Pharmacopoeia but prepared in the flower essence fashion – these are

mainly not covered in the FES repertory), and those which act mainly on the emotional plane, like the Bach remedies. It also has cross reference charts, rather than a repertory and a huge bibliography. Rather weighty in tone but essential for the serious student.

Healing Through Colour
Gimbel, Theo
Quantum

Form, Sound, Colour and Healing
Gimbel, Theo
Quantum

Colour Course
Steiner, Rudolph
Rudolph Steiner Press

Index

type remedy 58

Valerian 172, 189
verbal expressiveness 119
Vervain 35, 44–45
vibrational medicine 5–12,
    182
Vine 22, 23, 42, 45–46, 58
vital force 2

Walnut 46–47, 59
Waratah 144–45, 178
warmth 94, 110
water 6
Water Lily 180, 189
Water Violet 2, 47–48
Wedding Bush 145
Weeks, Nora 16
Welsh Poppy 172
White, Ian 73, 74, 121–22,
    124
White Bluebell 189
White Chestnut 48–49, 98,
    173
White Fireweed 161

White Spruce 161
White Violet 161
Wild Iris 189
Wild Oat 50–51
Wild Orchid 189
Wild Potato Bush 145
Wild Rhubarb 161
Wild Rose 51
Willow 45, 52, 161
Wisteria 145–46
Witch Hazel 172
Wood Anemone 172
work 86
worry 129

Yantra 187, 192
Yarrow 161
yearning 169
Yellow Cowslip Orchid 146
Yellow Dryas 161
Yellow Rattle 189
Yellow Silk Cotton Tree 180
Yerba Santa 120
Yew 173
Yorkshire Fog 173

HEALING HANDS
ALLEGRA TAYLOR

In this book, Allegra Taylor explores the potential we all possess to develop and channel our healing energies for the benefit of ourselves and our friends and family. Drawing on her experience as a practising healer, she dispels the myths surrounding healing and explains in a down to earth way the nature of the healing energy that surrounds us.

Many techniques – from crystals to visualization to aromatherapy – are detailed, along with practical guidelines to good health and wholeness.

THE BATES METHOD
PETER MANSFIELD

The Bates Method is a non-invasive and natural way of enhancing perception and relearning how to see, using simple and enjoyable techniques to relieve strain and improve brain/eye co-ordination.

Peter Mansfield, a practising Bates Method and Alexander Technique teacher, draws on a wide range of the therapeutic and educational experience in his introduction to this fascinating holistic approach to good sight.

ACUPUNCTURE
DR MICHAEL NIGHTINGALE
Acupuncture is a traditional Chinese therapy which usually (but not always) uses needles to stimulate the body's own energy and so bring healing. The author is a practising acupuncturist well aware of the particular concerns of first-time patients.

ALEXANDER TECHNIQUE
CHRIS STEVENS
Alexander Technique is a way of becoming more aware of balance, posture and movement in everyday activities. It can not only cure various complaints related to posture, such as backache, but teaches people to use their body more effectively and reduces stress.

AROMATHERAPY
GILL MARTIN
Aromatherapy uses the essential oils of plants, which are massaged into the skin, added to baths or taken internally to treat a variety of ailments and enhance general well-being.

ENCYCLOPAEDIA OF NATURAL MEDICINE
MICHAEL MURRAY and JOSEPH PIZZORNO

The Encyclopaedia of Natural Medicine is the most comprehensive guide and reference to the use of natural measures in the maintenance of good health and the prevention and treatment of disease. It explains the principles of natural medicine and outlines their application through the safe and effective use of herbs, vitamins, minerals, diet and nutritional supplements, and covers an extensive range of health conditions, from asthma to depression, from psoriasis to candidiasis, from diabetes to the common cold.

MEDITATION
ERICA SMITH and NICHOLAS WILKS

Meditation is a state of inner stillness which has been cultivated by mystics for thousands of years. The main reason for its recent popularity is that regular practice has been found to improve mental and physical health, largely due to its role in alleviating stress.

HYPNOSIS
URSULA MARKHAM

Hypnosis has a remarkable record of curing a wide range of ills. Ursula Markham, a practising hypnotherapist, explains how, by releasing inner tensions, hypnosis can help people to heal themselves.

CHIROPRACTIC
SUSAN MOORE

This guide to chiropractic concentrates on the actual treatment itself, seen from a patient's point of view. In a straightforward way, it answers all your questions about chiropractic, as well as providing background information about this popular therapy.

The author is a practising chiropractor, well aware of the concerns of first-time patients.

HERBAL MEDICINE
ANNE McINTYRE

Herbal medicine has been known for thousands of years. It is an entirely natural system of medicine which relies on the therapeutic quality of plants to enhance the body's recuperative powers, and so bring health – without any undesirable side effects.

MASSAGE THERAPY
ADAM JACKSON

A natural, safe and extremely effective therapy for everyone, it can be used as an aid to training in sport, in promoting healing after injury or as a relaxation technique. Message therapists work with footballers, weightlifters, athletes, alongside chiropractors and osteopaths, in hospitals or even assisting with the tensions in the boardroom.

IRIDOLOGY
ADAM JACKSON

Iridology is an ancient diagnostic technique through analysis of the iris of the eye. It is painless, non-invasive, and an astonishingly accurate method of health analysis which reveals the condition of each and every organ in the body. Iridologist Adam Jackson explains in a straightforward way how iridology works, what the basic markings and colours in the iris mean, and provides a guide to self-analysis.

He also outlines how to design a personal preventive healthcare programme using diet, exercise, stress management and natural therapies.

HEALING THE HEART
ELIZABETH WILDE McCORMICK

Every year in Britain 175,000 people survive heart attacks. But heart disease accounts for one in three deaths in the Western world and is the biggest killer in our society.

Drawing on recent, ongoing research into the effects of stress on the body, and the heart in particular, this book balances clinical fact with psychological considerations, linking mind, body and spirit. Taking a holistic approach, it explores how stress and unhappiness can harm the heart, and how underlying psychological issues have to be tackled along with the physical care of the heart.

SHIATSU
RAY RIDOLFI

This is a fascinating guide to the ancient art of Shiatsu.

Ray Ridolfi is a practising Shiatsu therapist and is well aware of the particular concerns of first-time patients. He has written a guide full of practical and straightforward advice as well as providing background information about this increasingly popular treatment.

[	] HEALING HANDS	£5.99
[	] THE BATES METHOD	£6.99
[	] ACUPUNCTURE	£6.99
[	] ALEXANDER TECHNIQUE	£6.99
[	] AROMATHERAPY	£6.99
[	] ENCYCLOPAEDIA OF NATURAL MEDICINE	£12.99
[	] MEDITATION	£6.99
[	] HYPNOSIS	£6.99
[	] CHIROPRACTIC	£6.99
[	] HERBAL MEDICINE	£6.99
[	] MASSAGE THERAPY	£6.99
[	] IRIDOLOGY	£6.99
[	] HEALING THE HEART	£6.99
[	] SHIATSU	£6.99

Optima Books now offers an exciting range of quality titles by both established and new authors which can be ordered from the following address:

Little, Brown and Company (UK),
P.O. Box 11, Falmouth, Cornwall TR10 9EN.
Alternatively you may fax your order to the above address. Fax No. 0326 376423.

Payments can be made as follows: cheque, postal order (payable to Little, Brown and Company) or by credit cards, Visa/Access. Do not send cash or currency. UK customers and B.F.P.O. please allow £1.00 for postage and packing for the first book, plus 50p for the second book, plus 30p for each additional book up to a maximum charge of £3.00 (7 books plus).

Overseas customers including Ireland please allow £2.00 for the first book plus £1.00 for the second book, plus 50p for each additional book.

NAME (Block Letters) ....

ADDRESS ....

I enclose my remittance for ....

I wish to pay by Access/Visa Card ....

Number ....

Card Expiry Date ....